The Tao of Chakras
On Living a Holistic Life

by

Daisy S. Zachariah MD

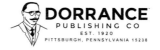

DORRANCE
PUBLISHING CO
EST. 1920
PITTSBURGH, PENNSYLVANIA 15238

Dorrance Publishing Co
585 Alpha Drive
Pittsburgh, PA 15238
Visit our website at *www.dorrancebookstore.com*

ISBN: 978-1-4809-4101-4
eISBN: 978-1-4809-4124-3

The Tao of Chakras
On Living a Holistic Life

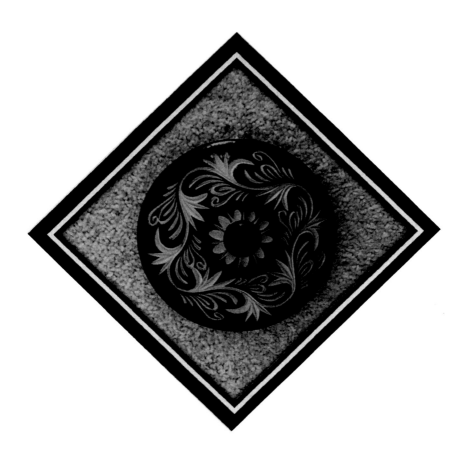

Cover illustration: This is a photograph of a piece of Malaysian pottery. The photograph is taken with deliberate imperfection.

An imperfection is deliberately woven into the corner of a Persian rug. This practice of intentionally including an irregularity is honoring the religious belief that god is the only perfect being. This perfection-in-imperfection is also seen in Navajo rugs. The Navajo say this is "where the spirit moves in and out of the rug." Native American beadwork always has an intentional flaw to show that the artisan was human. An asymmetric flaw was also common in Gothic or Romanesque architecture. Our lives are never perfect but it is beautiful nevertheless.

The central core in the image, is stable and solid, crafted with beauty; as so is our central core.

The circular whorl symbolizes the vortex of chakras and the cycle of life. Life is never an even, smooth circle but side tracks with pitfalls, spectacular explosions and colorful adornments. Back on the wheel of life we are richer for the experience if we choose to make it so.

The image is enclosed in a diamond, a most precious gem, known for its sparkle and hardness. Diamonds are formed deep in earth's mantle about 150 km below the earth's crust. It takes time for diamonds to form from carbon, requiring very high pressures and temperatures of over 1000 degrees Celsius. Carbon, the same element that is in a lump of coal, undergoes change to manifest its amazing potential of beauty and strength.

Our lives can sparkle brilliantly if we allow the transformation through the tough principles laid out in the Tao (wisdom) of the Chakras.

This
Book is
Dedicated
To
My children three
Jason, Janis, Jaime

Love of my life
Sculptor
of
my
Soul

CONTENTS

Illustrations of the brain

PREFACE

"The purpose of life is not to be happy. It is to be useful, to be honorable, to be compassionate, to have it make some difference that you have lived and lived well."
—Ralph Waldo Emerson

We are immersed in a society of poverty, discrimination, and social inequities. Daily reports of mass shootings, political unrest, international terrorism, and wars assault our senses through the media. We fight violence with violence, hoping to bring about the peace we so deeply crave. Depression, suicide, and addictions run rampant in our society today. There is no doubt that there is a dire need for change—a change to effect peace and cooperation and to live in alignment with our environment and the cosmos.

Every religion can boast of believers who have made a positive impact in this world. By the same token, many famous people have excelled in one sphere but failed in other aspects. Presidents have fallen, brought down by sexual indiscretion or intrigue. "Upright" catholic clergy have shamed the institution with their debauchery and sexual misdeeds. Film stars adored by the public end up with drug overdose and suicidal deaths. There is a character disconnect that seems to be the human condition.

Sometimes we question if we have any control over our lives and whether fate runs our lives. But fate or nature is a default mode. We can change and influence the course of events in our lives and ultimately the planet.

In our world of imposed rules and regulations, inequalities and injustices, and the resulting suffering, change has to come one person at a time. Change has to start with "ME" —*the (wo)man in the mirror*. Change has to come from within. With this change comes personal health and happiness diffusing into meaningful change in this amazing world we live in.

Gandhi encourages us to be *the change we wish to see in the world*. If we wish to eradicate all that causes or threatens discord, we must radiate random acts of kindness and gratitude. Having this dedicated sense of purpose with tolerance to alternate world views will break down barriers of suspicion and mistrust.

As we explore the concepts outlined here and understand ourselves better, we can effect change and bloom right where we are. Life need not be a reactive struggle to win or defeat. Life is a celebration of one's identity.

We no longer hold the ancient belief that disease was caused by demonic influences. The importance of diet, lifestyle, emotions, and environment are undisputed. Yet we often sabotage ourselves and revert to unhealthy habits of living. The brain, in its default network, favors well-worn neural pathways or habits. Breaking these habits is possible. New ways of thinking and behaving can be learned as the brain is capable of creating new patterns of neural connections. This scientific term for this is neuroplasticity. Change can be small, one step at a time. Also we are finding, through genetic and epigenetic studies, that genes can change and that what we are is not fixed or carved in stone.

Taking positive steps and finding pleasure in what we do leads to dopamine release, increasing energy and drive. Being able to step back from negative or stressful thoughts can change our perception of reality. We can train ourselves to seek a life of true happiness, compassion and empathy. We can change old ways of thinking and form neural pathways to encourage and promote harmony and the common good. As we understand and appreciate our reality, we move towards positive growth. Every affirmative choice of letting go of fear, distrust, and anger adds to the positive "mood" of this planet from hatred and violence to love and peace.

Understanding and defining our needs and boundaries allows us to communicate that to those around us. With purposeful living, conscious of the common good, we can live each day with courage and compassion speckled with a pinch of humor. We can strive to be attentive to our inner wisdom using the tools we are given. We have to be motivated to make this change. The path may be rough and rocky; there may be heartbreak and tears. The reward is the promise of a life more beautiful than ever dreamed of.

Self-study and self-cultivation are the keys to becoming more than we were before. The practice of focused awareness and attention provides the entry.

As we work on ourselves, we not only change the mood around us, we change the way we are perceived. As we smile from the inside out, the "smile" is dispersed like a ripple from a stone thrown in the sea. Our smile reflects back to us. This work we do, when intrinsically motivated, rather than as a result of external pressures or self-aggrandizement, becomes rewarding and life giving.

I have adapted the basic schema of the ancient Hindu Chakras system, for self-study and change; giving it a down to earth interpretation without the mysticism. Using the Chakra system as a visual illustration, I have organized aspects of our lives in a systematic format to bring cohesiveness to the spectrum of healthy living. I also weave in neurobiological considerations, current medical applications of general interest and relevance as well as meditative exercises. Charts and photographs and are included for clarification and interest.

My sources for the book are drawn from my medical training and experience, Hindu and Buddhist writings, ancient myths and traditions from all cultures, as well as current scientific facts.

Considering the scope of this enterprise, I have merely touched on the essentials for personal and global health and happiness. The concepts in this book, although challenging to live up to, will impact your life and the lives of others. While on our path to wholeness, we may be buffeted like the waves on the sea and have our hearts broken. Like Sisyphus, our stone might keep rolling back but we must push on till the tipping point is reached. The health of humanity and the planet depends on it.

This book is by no means a comprehensive manual for living as knowledge will change over time, nor is it meant to replace advice from your personal physician. My hope is that between the pages of this book, you may find a nugget or two that speaks to you. *The Tao of Chakras: On Living a Holistic Life* is meant to be thought-provoking. It is not exclusive of other opinions. Not being a scholar in chakra philosophy or the Vedas, I honor the beliefs of others who have found meaning in the mystical interpretations of the chakras.

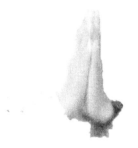

INTRODUCTION TO THE CHAKRAS

Before written language, education was oral and handed down by the sages. In India, ancient wisdom was first recorded on palm leaves and has been modified and added to as the Vedas—the Hindu text of knowledge. The chakras are first mentioned in these Vedic texts. The chakra system was elaborated further in the Upanishads as psychic centers of consciousness and is integrally linked to yoga philosophy. According to the writer, Anodea Judith, in the book *Wheel of life*, these writings are traced back to the Aryans who invaded India in the second century BCE and brought with them their culture and myths.

Currently, there is a vast amount of literature relating to the Chakra system and its meaning, not always consistent or universal. However, the basic tenets remain similar. Although the chakra centers have been interpreted to occupy physical locations in the body, there probably were layers of allegorical meaning added to, and expanded on, over time.

In brief, the Chakras are believed to be vortices of energy depicted as seven circles or lotuses located along the spine. The Sanskrit term chakra means wheel or circle, possibly referring to the wheels of the chariots of the invading Aryans or possibly the circle of time or the disc of the sun. When the chakras are awakened (becoming aware of) they "open up like flowers (or lotuses) and pour out their qualities" establishing inner balance and harmony.

The concept of energy centers is not isolated to Vedic literature. The Hopi Indians believe that all mankind is fashioned by the Creator with five "vibratory centers" located at various points along the vertebral column which are used as a means of communication with the universe and the Creator. This communication is accomplished by gentle vibrations which resonate from these five corporeal points. The first of these points is the "Kopavi," meaning "open door" which is the soft spot on the head of a newborn child. It is believed that at the time of death, life exits the body through the Kopavi just as it entered it at birth. The Chinese concept of the vital energy of the Universe or "Chi" flows through pathways in the body as known as meridians. This energy is at the foundation of many health and fitness practices such as Tai Chi, Martial Arts, and Reiki.

As in Jewish "Midrash," where stories can be experienced or understood at multiple levels, the chakras have multiple levels of meaning. This might explain the variations seen in the literature. The chakras traditionally are associated with various mantras, deities, mystical significance, organs in the body and aspects of self.

The ancients used what was around them as sources of inspiration and a means for instruction. Each energy circle is associated with a specific color, sound, and fixed number of petals. Isaac Newton chose seven colors in his description of the visible spectrum of light because that was the number of notes in the musical scale, which he believed was related to the optical spectrum. Newton included indigo, the hue between blue and violet, as one of the separate colors of the spectrum of light. Today it is usually considered a hue of blue resulting in six colors of the rainbow. The colors of the vortices are ascribed to these 6 colors of the rainbow, red for the first chakra, violet for the sixth; white for the seventh chakra, an amalgamation of the six colors.

The number of petals progresses from four at the root chakra to a thousand petals at the crown chakra. The number of petals are apparently related to bones/vertebrae associated with each of the chakras except the crown chakra. Being an oral tradition, it is possible that the number of petals was used as a means to pass down knowledge much as counting on fingers or repeating the rosary.

Using current anatomical knowledge I postulate that the four bones of the pelvis, the ischium, ilium, pubis and coccyx correlate to the four petals for the first chakra; the five lumbar vertebrae with the sacrum are the six petals for second chakra; the ten ribs for the third chakra (the eleventh and twelfth ribs being rudimentary and not attached to the sternum may have been viewed as part of the vertebra); and twelve thoracic vertebrae for the fourth chakra.

The four bones (or cartilages) of the larynx, the three bones of the sternum (or breast bone), the clavicle, the maxilla (or jaw bone) and the seven cervical (neck) vertebrae correlates to the sixteen petals for the fifth (throat) chakra.

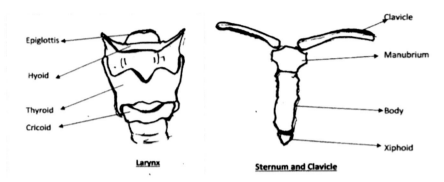

Epiglottis

Hyoid

Thyroid

Cricoid

Larynx

Clavicle

Manubrium

Body

Xiphoid

Sternum and Clavicle

The two petals of the sixth chakra can be said to relate to the two halves of the skull or cerebrum.

In the human body, there is the central nervous system (brain and spinal cord) and the autonomic nervous system. The central nervous system links with the peripheral nervous system to allow input of sensory impulses from the environment and action (motor) output for activities of the body. The autonomic nervous system (ANS) is the internal sensor for the body connecting the body to brain. It's excitatory or sympathetic and the inhibitory or parasympathetic components function as checks and balances like the accelerator and the brakes of a car.

These nerves (together with the peripheral nerves) form networks known as plexuses along the spine. It is conceivable, in ancient times, that these nerve plexuses with its complex whorls gave rise to the concept of the chakras.

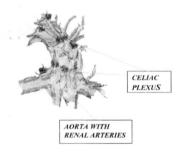

CELIAC PLEXUS

AORTA WITH RENAL ARTERIES

Modifying the traditional interpretation of the chakras, I elaborate the format of the chakras to bring a healthy understanding of our lives.

Visualize arms and legs as mere extensions of the body. The base then sits at the bottom of the spine. This is the natural "root" of the body which ancient wisdom called the root chakra. It corresponds to the group of nerves exiting from the base of the spinal canal like the roots of a tree. The first chakra governs the essential core needs and functions of the body.

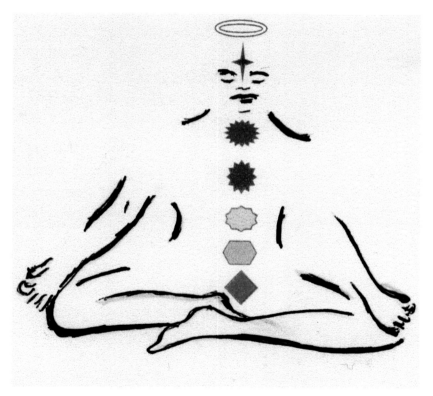

The sacral chakra locates at the sacral plexus and relates to the senses, pleasure, and sexual organs. This chakra is also known as the swadisthana or "seat of self. Identification with one's sexuality is prevalent in all communities. Many jokes are made about males "thinking with their gonads." Similarly women's behaviors and mood swings are associated with the ovulation and/or menstruation.

The third chakra is located at the solar (coeliac) plexus or the pit of the stomach and relates to the emotions. Colloquially, we say "it grabs you in the pit of the stomach," or I "feel butterflies in my stomach." In their wisdom, the ancients have called this center the "city of gems," as they recognize the power of the emotions and its potential when harnessed.

The fourth chakra, corresponding to the cardiac plexus, is the heart chakra where a different force that governs life is situated. This is a force of selfless love, compassion, and virtues. Unlike the lower three chakras that follow the laws that govern nature (as in animals and lower life forms) this chakra is directed by will and choice.

The fifth chakra, the throat chakra, is assigned to the throat or voice box, and is representative of expression and truth. It corresponds to the pharyngeal plexus and branches from the vagus nerve that innervate the voice box.

The sixth chakra or "third eye" chakra centered between the eyebrows, traditionally is the center for intuition and wisdom. It corresponds to the pineal gland. I have interpreted this as the center for consciousness.

The seventh or crown chakra symbolizes detachment from illusion and the oneness of all. Often referred to as "a thousand petaled lotus" it is the state of divine bliss or Samadhi in the ancient texts. It is the merger of the six chakras just as white comprises all the six colors of the rainbow. The chakra centers, in the ancient writings, are interconnected by two snakes or spirals traversing the spine. Human characteristics depicted by the chakras, are all interrelated and assume equal importance. Hence, this chakra is the state of complete integration.

The lotus flower has much symbolic meaning in Egyptian, Hindu, and Buddhist cultures. The beautiful lotus flower arises out of murky, muddy waters. Rising and blooming above the murky waters has been an analogy for enlightenment and /or purification. The petals of the lotus flower open during the day and close at night, symbolizing cycles of day and night, birth and rebirth. Taken in figurative sense, rebirth signifies a change of ideas or rising from a dark period in life. The strong stem of the lotus pushing its way out of the mud and against strong currents, depicts strength.

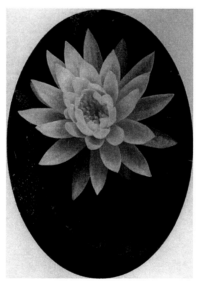

The fully bloomed lotus with its seated Buddha, signifies strength of character, transcending earthly pleasures to reach enlightenment.

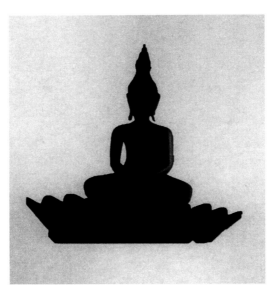

Using the framework of the chakra system as a tool for self-knowledge and awareness, based on current science and understanding, we can rise above our dark, murky waters to bloom and reach our full potential and attain maximum health and happiness.

Reframing my interpretation of the chakras in a graphic illustration we have the Wheel or Spokes for Holistic Living as seen below:

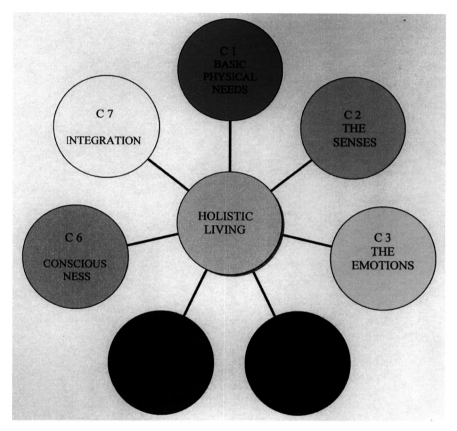

Spokes for Holistic Living

CHAKRA 1

THE ROOT CHAKRA
FOUR PETALS OF BASIC NEEDS

SLEEP
Rest & Relaxation

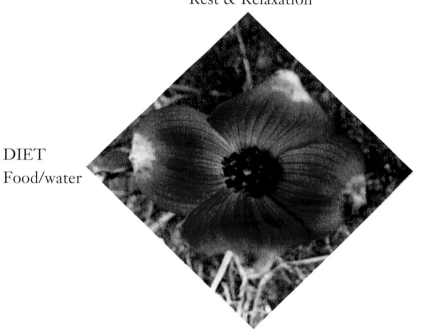

DIET
Food/water

EXERCISE
Activity

BREATH
Air

Chapter 1
FOUR PETALS OF BASIC NEEDS

"To keep the body in good health is a duty...otherwise
we shall not be able to keep the mind strong and clear"
—Buddha

Since ancient times it has been known that taking care of the basic needs of the body equates to optimum health. In Greek mythology, around the sixth or seventh century BC, Asclepius, the son of Apollo and Coronis, was a Greek hero who later became the Greek god of Medicine and Healing. His legacy lives on in the modern medical symbol of staff and snake. Long after his death, the temples of Asclepius carried on his teachings of healing in the form of diet, rest, massage, hydrotherapy and religion. Because he was said to cure the sick in dreams, the supplicants for healing slept in the temples. Here they were exposed to soothing music and healing spas. They waited for Asclepius to visit and give them advice on diet, baths and exercise.

Pythagoras and his followers formed a school of philosophy and religious teachings extolling purity of mind and behavior and promoting the virtues of a frugal vegetarian diet. The main Pythagorean therapy was diet, exercise, music and meditation. Cabbage and anise were recommended to maintain health and treat illness.

The year 460 BC celebrated the birth of Hippocrates, the Father of Medicine. He was exposed to the above philosophies of healing through the Asclepion temple in Cos where he grew up. Hippocrates based his practice on observations and study of the body. He believed that illness had a physical and rational explanation and rejected the view that illness was caused by the disfavor of gods or possession by evil spirits, which was the prevalent thinking of the times. He taught the prevention of disease through diet and exercise, fresh air and cleanliness. He taught that the body contains within itself the power to heal, *"our natures are the physicians of our disease."* Therapy was to augment or facilitate this natural process. This principle holds true today.

The ancient Egyptians also understood the need for proper diet and exercise, emphasizing only the consumption of natural and healthy foods. They recognized that illness was a sign of internal turmoil.

The first requirement of a new born baby is to breathe. Sleep and rest come next. Soon after, the infant needs feeding and movement (exercise). These basic functions provide all of baby's physical needs; these needs continue throughout life.

Breath is the mechanism for obtaining oxygen which is essential to human life—there is no life without breath. Aborigines of Australia heal headaches by blowing their breath across the patient's head to remove a foreign spirit or "mamu." This is followed by neck massage and the manipulation of 'strings' believed to control the blood flow to the brain. We still see parents blowing on a child's "owie" to make it better.

Yoga and Tai Chi focus on breath, mindful movement and low-impact exercises with proven physical and mental health benefits. Native Americans in Arizona run each day to greet the dawn, a practice that not only conditions their bodies but also nourishes their spiritual wellbeing. Massage, Reiki, and spa treatments have been used throughout centuries attesting the benefits of rest and relaxation to health.

Studies show the importance of getting the recommended six to eight hours of sleep a night. Insufficient sleep is linked with mood disorders, heart disease and sudden death.

We eat to live. Life ends without food (and water) for nourishment and growth. Eastern and aboriginal philosophies have a concept of hot and cold foods that are used to balance and heal the body. In Aboriginal Australia, Africa and India, native plants are used as medicine. Herbal therapies and living in harmony with the earth are very much a part of indigenous cultures. Today herbs and foods that are rich in "antioxidants" are widely promoted. Alternative medical practitioners use a wide variety of treatments ranging from herbs, fasting and dieting to toxic cleanses and massage.

The ancient Hindu system of healing known as Ayurveda recognizes that the two main areas that affect health are diet and lifestyle. According to Ayurveda, there are six stages of disease. First is the initial exposure to an injury, neglect or a toxin. Repeated insults lead to accumulation of toxin which then spreads throughout the body and concentrates at a specific site or organ. As a result we become ill. With continued insults organ tissue is irreparably damaged and chronic disease and organ failure occurs. With this explanation we can appreciate why chronic diseases such as diabetes and hypertension occur. Repeated damage to the body by poor diet and an unhealthy lifestyle over time leads to chronic disease.

In modern medicine there is overwhelming data that corroborates the claims of the ancient healers and show that diet and lifestyle are major determinants of health and wellness. If we took a number of people with heart attacks or strokes and traced their lives back, we would find that a large majority would have had poor diets and tended to be sedentary. A poor lifestyle led to high cholesterol, diabetes and hypertension and eventually stroke, heart attack and premature death.

Thus we see that the basic tenets for health have remained consistent throughout the ages. Oxygen (the breath), diet, exercise and sleep form the foundation or pillars for health. The definition of foundation is *"the underlying base or support upon which something is built."* These four core fundamentals for wellness are the four petals for The Root Chakra in my schema. A strong root supports the mighty tree keeping it stable in the face of winds and storms.

These basic needs are directed by the reptilian brain or the brain stem. The reptilian brain orchestrates the essential functions of the body such as feeding and breathing. This reptilian brain evolved, over time, to form the mid brain and the limbic system to interact with the external world and generate and modulate emotion. This evolved brain, found in the animal kingdom is the mammalian brain. It is with the development of the neocortex, the complex human brain, that higher level thinking and orchestration became possible.

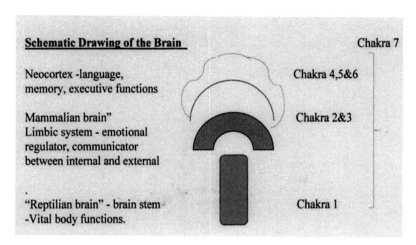

Schematic Drawing of the Brain

Neocortex -language, memory, executive functions

Mammalian brain" Limbic system - emotional regulator, communicator between internal and external

"Reptilian brain" - brain stem -Vital body functions.

Chakra 7

Chakra 4,5&6

Chakra 2&3

Chakra 1

Traditionally, the root chakra is described as being "at the base of the spine." I have assigned it to the pelvic floor—the diamond shaped area bounded by the seat bones (or the ischial tuberosities) on both sides, the coccyx or tail bone behind and the pubic symphysis or midline joint between the pubic bones in front. Just like a four legged stool, it represents the base or foundation, a visual representation of grounding and stability upon which the pillars of wellness are built.

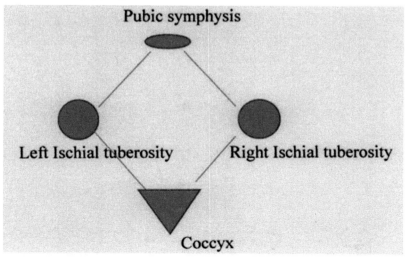

Pubic symphysis

Left Ischial tuberosity

Right Ischial tuberosity

Coccyx

The color for the root Chakra is red. Red is the color at the end of the spectrum of visible light. It is one of the three primary colors reflecting its importance. It is the color of life's blood and the precious gemstones, garnet and ruby. It signifies power and commands attention. Alert signs and signals for stop and danger are usually in red. Stop to give due consideration to the four pillars of health on a daily basis.

The following chapters expand on these fundamental needs for wellness and human flourishing—the breath, sleep, diet, and exercise.

Chapter 2
BREATH OF LIFE

And the Lord God formed man of the dust of the ground, and breathed into his nostrils the breath of life; and man became a living soul.

—Genesis 2:7 kjv

"I am never alone wherever I am. The air itself supplies me with a century of love. When I breathe in, I am breathing in the laughter, tears, victories, passions, thoughts, memories, existence, joys, moments, and the hues of the sunlight on many tones of skin; I am breathing in the same air that was exhaled by many before me. The air that bore them life. And so how can I ever say that I am alone?"

—C. JoyBell C.

Breath is the essence of life. To determine if a person is dead or alive, we check the breath. If the windpipe is blocked for any length of time by a bolus of food, by choking or drowning, life is terminated. Blockage of an oxygen-rich artery with a clot cuts off the oxygen supply and leads to death of the tissue supplied by that artery. When that happens to the heart muscle, we call it a heart attack. And when it occurs in the brain, we call it a brain attack or stroke.

We live in a sea of air much as a fish lives in an ocean of water. The soul of the universe fills us with each breath we take. Oxygen, from the air we breathe, travels down the windpipe or trachea to the bronchial tubes and the alveolar sacs of the lungs. From here the oxygen diffuses across the membranes into the blood stream where it is taken up by the red blood cells. From the blood stream, the oxygen from the red blood cells moves into every cell of the body. Oxygen is the energy source used for growth, repair and formation of new cells. The metabolic processes in the cell lead to waste in the form of carbon dioxide and water. These are transported back to the bloodstream, then to the lungs and breathed back into the atmosphere. This cycle of taking in oxygen and releasing carbon dioxide is, amazingly, reversed in plant life which takes in carbon dioxide and releases oxygen during photosynthesis. The animal and plant kingdoms sustain each other in a delicate balance.

From the first breath the baby takes at the time of delivery till the last breath of the dying, breathing is a natural, rhythmic, involuntary process. It is the first source of energy to the body. Although breathing is natural it remains unconscious for the most part, directed by the brain stem or primitive brain.

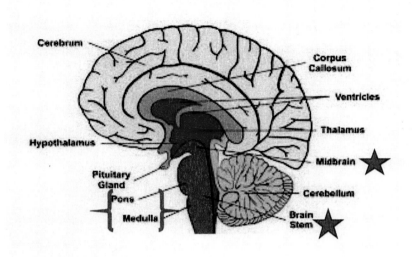

Mid brain and Brainstem
Adapted from Wikimedia commons
http://medicalndex.com/human-brain-anatomy-inside-skull-2

The areas identified as the medulla and the pons in the brain stem regulate our breathing. Involuntary rhythmic nerve impulses from these centers activate and contract to relax the muscles of the diaphragm and ribs and cause inspiration and expiration to occur. The respiration rate is modulated by the level of oxygen and carbon dioxide in the blood. This forms a feedback loop that keeps the oxygen level at a steady state. There is a fine balance in the different components regulating our breath without awareness on our part. Respiration can however be modified by emotions, activity and changes in temperature. We also have the ability to control our breathing if and when we choose, by the higher cortical centers through the vagus nerve, which is part of the autonomic nervous system.

Breathing is the heart of all meditative practices. It deepens awareness, decreases emotional fluctuations and expands consciousness. Breath and life's energy are one. The yogis or wise men of the East, call this energy "prana," and the Chinese call it "chi." "Pranayama," or "breath control," uses the breath to affect the physical, emotional and spiritual body. According to the yogis, breath can be retrained and directed into subtle energy channels, called "nadis," which in turn activates the energy centers of the chakras.

The ancient writings of the Vedas and the Taoist Canon, the Tao Tsang, describes in great detail the myriad ways one can harness the energy of the breath. Breath is described as the handle to gain control of one's mind and body. The writings of Lao Tzu written centuries ago detail how the breathing is to be refined and trained and the secret exercises that might prolong life.

Tibetan monks engage in a deep meditative trance through breath control and intent by which they are able to warm up a wet sheet wrapped around themselves in the heart of winter. This practice known as ptumo (or tummo) illustrates the power of conscious breath.

A simple experiment to validate this, is to use a basal body thermometer which registers very small increments in body heat. Hold the thermometer between thumb and first two fingers firmly. By consciously directing breath to the fingers notice the increase in the temperature of the finger tips.

Deep, conscious breathing and full expansion of the lungs is a powerfully energizing tool. Physiologically, as more oxygen is distributed to the tissues, all cellular functions are enhanced to better repair, detoxify and combat disease. Optimally nourished cells make for a healthier body.

Medical Applications

Breathing fresh clean air is an important part of health. Chemical pollutants, such as cigarette smoke, and toxic chemical vapors reduce the availability of oxygen and harms the natural processes of the body.

As we age, the microcirculation of our organs and tissues deteriorates. Narrowing of the arteries reduces oxygenation and thereby contributes to strokes and heart attacks. Breathing exercises help to open these channels and improve microcirculation. Multiple sub-clinical episodes of disruption of blood flow to the brain constricts and reduces the flow of oxygen. This leads to what is known as multi-infarct dementia or vascular dementia. It is conceivable that conscious breathing with intent, visualizing blood flow to the brain may delay or minimize this degenerative process.

With an acute exacerbation or acute attack of asthma, the bronchial tubes constrict reducing air flow. With breathing exercises, we utilize more of the reserve lung function and minimize the severity of an asthma attack. The same holds true for other lung impairments such as chronic obstructive lung disease (COPD).

Breathing exercises are anti-aging as it preserves respiratory muscle functions, lubricates the rib joints and maintains optimal lung function. As we grow older, there is decreased ability of the chest wall to expand and contract both from calcification at the rib joints and progressive weakness of the chest wall muscles. Breathing exercises lubricates the rib joints and strengthens the intercostal muscles. With aging there is decreased elastic recoil, resulting in collapse of the lung tissue. Breathing exercises helps to expand the lungs, open the areas of collapsed lung tissue and increase the mean ventilation volume.

There is a correlation between emotional states and the breath. The mind and the breath are interrelated. With fear and anxiety, the breath is shallow and rapid. By conscious breathing, we activate the vagus nerve to release a neurotransmitter or chemical called acetylcholine which decreases heart rate and blood pressure, reducing anxiety and inducing calm. Conscious breathing may also play a role in treating depression, and panic attacks. The use and dose of medications and its concomitant side effects for these crippling mental problems can be reduced by bringing awareness to the breath.

Another unexpected research finding is that controlled breathing can alter the expression of genes involved in immune function, energy metabolism and insulin secretion. The study for these findings was co-authored by Dr. Herbert Benson.

Meditative Exercise
Sit comfortably, either on a chair or cross-legged on a cushion or the floor, and focus on breathing. Allow the in-breath to expand the lungs using abdominal breathing. This is the way that babies breathe. With each inspiration the abdomen and lower ribs expands outwards and with each expiration the abdomen and rib cage contracts. The lung tissue expands maximally with each in breath. Areas that are generally collapsed are expanded with each slow, deep and full breath. So fewer breaths are needed to supply the body with life-giving oxygen, conserving energy and relaxing the body.

The breath should not be forced. Breathing should be like the tide; gentle with the in-flow and relaxed with the out-flow. Let your breathing be steady and even. Breathe in through the nostrils to filter and warm the air. Mentally count to five as you breathe in and count to five as you breathe out. Work on gradually increasing the count to seven for the out-breath.

As you focus on the breathing, notice that the mind quietens and cluttered extraneous thoughts are reduced. Visualizing the breath as peace adds to the calming effect. Visualizing each breath flowing to each organ gives a greater awareness of the body and increases its blood supply.

As your mind quietens acknowledge your place in the universe, and the interconnection between all living things. Plant and animal life sustains each other with a natural synergy in the universe. The air we breathe is the link.

With this daily practice of harnessing the breath, comes clarity of mind, enhancement of the physical body, and calmness of spirit.

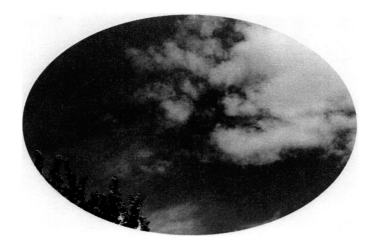

Tacoma, WA

Chapter 3
REST AND SLEEP

"Don't fight with the pillow, but lay down your head
And kick every worriment out of the bed."
—Edmund Vance Cooke

In the Bible, the first act of creation was the formation of light, dividing it from darkness, setting the stage for a time to be awake and a time for sleep. The Egyptian myth of creation tells that in the beginning there was only the dark, swirling watery chaos, called Nu. Out of these chaotic waters rose Atum, the sun god. His emergence can be interpreted as the coming of light into the darkness.

In Greek mythology, the awareness of the power of sleep is depicted by Hypnos, god of sleep and child of Nyx (darkness). Hypnos was depicted as gentle and mild; yet had power over all gods, mortals and animals. His task was to roam the world to relieve people of worries and pains. The Blackfoot Indians visualize sleep as a gentle, soft butterfly. Blackfoot women embroider a butterfly on buckskin and tie it into baby's hair. They sing lullabies of a butterfly coming to bring sleep to the baby. Mr. Sandman, a children's fantasy or folk figure, creeps into the bedroom at night and drops his magic sand on children giving them beautiful dreams. This fable is probably the source for the phrase "morning sand in my eye."

Sleep has been the focus of much poetry and prose and has been called Father of dreams, master of the unconscious and liberator of daily chores. Sleep is a natural pause in life's daily activity—a transition from the outer life to the inner workings of the mind and body.

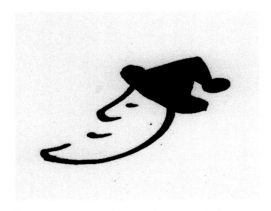

Much has been written about sleep and dreaming. Carl Jung, a psychologist, believed that dreams are the shortcut to the unconscious and has written much about the significance and the interpretation of dreams.

Nothing seems to be more natural than sleep, yet it is still an activity shrouded in mystery. Considering that we spend thirty percent of our lives sleeping, we need to respect that there is more to sleep than meets the eye. In recent times science has brought some understanding to sleep and sleep disorders and the impact sleep has on health and well-being.

The body is a fine tuned machine guided by Circadian rhythms. These daily rhythms, or internal clocks regulate the sleep-wake cycle. The sleep-wake system is regulated by the synchronization of processes that promote sleep and maintain wakefulness. Photoreceptor nerve cells in the retina of the eye detect the level of light/dark and sends this information to the suprachiasmatic nucleus, responsible for controlling circadian rhythms. This in turn stimulates the pineal gland to secrete melatonin which induces sleepiness. Secretion of melatonin is maximum at night and falls during the day in response to the light. The sleep-generating system also influences neurons in the pons (upper brain stem). These neurons send outputs to the lower brainstem and spinal cord to cause loss of muscle tone and slowing of the heart rate that occurs during sleep.

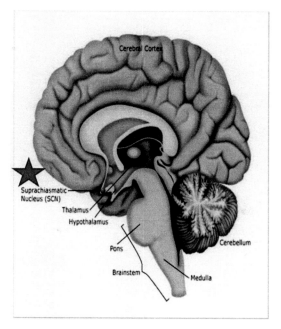

Adapted from creative commons licensed under CC- BY SA 4.0

In general adults need about six to eight hours of sleep a night. With brain wave studies it has been found that normal sleep consists of REM (rapid eye movement) sleep and three stages of light to deep non REM sleep. The different stages seem to cycle in about ninety minute stretches. REM sleep generally occurs about four to five times a night and occupies twenty percent of sleep time. REM sleep tends to increase when there has been stress, emotionally charged events or major life crises during the day. Apparently this brain activity during sleep sorts, integrates and consolidates memory amongst other restorative, physiological functions. REM sleep is the period of sleep where dreaming occurs.

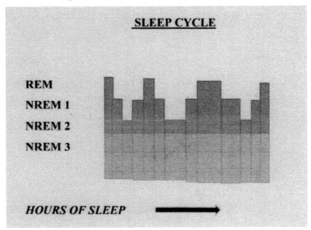

The analogy for sleep is that of a computer shutting down or rebooting; or a battery recharging. Sleep is a state of consciousness where the brain is less conscious of external happenings and becomes tuned in to the internal workings of the body. Many restorative functions of the body occur during the time of sleep. The core temperature decreases, muscles are relaxed, heart rate drops and blood pressure lowers. Apparently sleep washes out the byproducts and toxins of neural activity accumulated during the day and restores healthy brain chemicals. Prescription medications and alcohol may help a person to get to sleep but the quality of sleep and the restorative functions of REM sleep are diminished.

These same bodily changes that occur with sleep are seen with rest and meditation. The essence of meditation is to train the mind to shut off external stimuli as well as decrease the endless chatter in the brain. Meditation gives us much needed rest from our busy schedules and life's daily stresses. Meditative techniques train us to focus on one thing such as the breath, or a word (mantra) turning off the flow of thought. This brings about a relaxation response leading to a lowered heart rate, blood pressure and muscle tension. It has been claimed that twenty minutes of meditation is as good as a full night's sleep. Although often thought of as **a** Buddhist practice, meditation is at the heart of many spiritual practices and can be practiced without any religious overtones. It is a way of self-understanding and healing. The mindfulness meditation program at the Massachusetts stress reduction clinic has shown proven health benefits in patients with chronic illness. Long term meditators also have claimed improved memory, creativity and alertness.

Medical Applications

Sleep is essential for life. Sleep deprivation is known to lead to difficulty in focusing, irritability and aggression. Just observe a child who missed his afternoon nap! Patients with sleep disturbances often present with headaches, depression and anxiety. There is a decrease in cognitive functions as well. Hand/eye coordination in the sleep deprived is impaired and speed and accuracy of tasks suffer. Sleep deprivation leads to daytime drowsiness. Falling asleep at the wheel has been associated with road traffic accidents and statistically matches alcohol related accidents. Poor sleep translates into poor work performance and quality of social relationships. Fibromyalgia and musculoskeletal aches and pains are associated with poor sleep. Immune functions are impaired and there is an associated increase in cardiovascular disease.

Patients who suffer from sleep apnea (abnormally long pause in breathing during sleep) may be at greater risk for sudden death. With the prolonged apneic episode, the oxygen level falls to dangerously low levels; irregular heart rhythms or a lowered heart rate occur leading to sudden death. The repetitive episodes of hypoxia (low oxygen) are thought to trigger cellular and biochemical processes which predispose to atherosclerosis or hardening of the arteries. Multiple arousals which occur with sleep apnea are associated with hypertension. Patients with sleep apnea are more likely to have the metabolic syndrome with weight and blood pressure issues.

Too much of a good thing is just as harmful for the body and excessive sleep (more than nine hours a night on a consistent basis) translates to sluggishness, obesity and a higher risk of diabetes, heart disease and depression.

Substance abusers exhibit disrupted sleep /wake rhythms. People who travel between time zones experience jet lag as their internal clock is scrambled, with symptoms of fatigue, disorientation, and insomnia. Shift workers experience similar symptoms for the same reasons.

Meditative Exercise

It is important in our busy, frenzied schedules to take time to relax, recharge and rejuvenate. The world keeps on turning, even if you take time off for yourself.

Lay on a grassy field in summer and watch the clouds drift by. Take a walk by the ocean and listen to the tide as it gently laps the sandy beaches. Hike up a trail in the mountains and notice the foliage around you.

As with all other life aspects, knowledge is power. Knowing the importance of sleep, indulge yourself around bedtime. Take a languid bath/shower so the body is refreshed and relaxed. Maintain a relaxing atmosphere with soft music and low lighting. Keep the temperature comfortable. Have fresh clean sheets that feel sensuous and luxurious. Settle in bed feeling the softness and the support the bed has to offer.

Gently breathe into your abdomen, breathing in peace and breathing out peace to surround you as in chapter two. Consciously focus on each part of your body in turn. Relax your toes, ankles, calves and thighs in turn. Release the tension in the buttock and abdomen. Loosen up your fingers, arms and shoulders. Feel the rhythmic beat of your heart and the gentle rise and fall of your chest with each breath. Relax your throat and neck. Release the lower jaw and let the tongue rest gently on the upper palate. Relax your eyes and forehead. Experience the softening and letting go of all tension in your body and mind. Drift off into your own special place of calm and serenity.

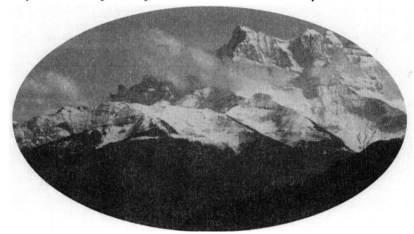

Pre Alps Lake Geneva

Chapter 4
FOOD FOR LIFE

"From earth herbs, from herbs food, from food seed, from seed man. Man thus consists of the essence of food"
—Upanishad

"When you rise in the morning, give thanks for the light, for your life, for your strength. Give thanks for your food and for the joy of living."
—Tecumseh

Hippocrates, the Father of Medicine, wrote 2,500 years ago, *"Let your food be your medicine."* Food is a basic human need and a source of energy for all living things. In humans, food has come to mean much more than mere sustenance.

Food is the center of social activity and pleasure, the simple meal being the focus of a family gathering and sharing. Thanksgiving dinner, in celebration of the harvest, is often a family or community affair. Weddings and birthdays gather friends and family to mark the special occasion, and its significance with special feasts.

Food is often symbolic. The Jewish Seder during Passover observes the exodus from Egypt during the reign of Ramses II and freedom from slavery. The Seder Meal is elaborate with customs and remembrances. The Seder plate consists of five foods: three pieces of matzo (unleavened bread being used to signify the haste with which the Israelites had to leave Egypt). Parsley dipped in salt water expresses tears of the people. A roasted egg marks new beginnings. A shank bone symbolizes the sacrificial offering. And lastly, bitter herbs evoke the bitter affliction of slavery. The last Supper was actually a Seder meal but is passed on in the Christian tradition as the Holy Communion.

Food as a sacrifice is common to all religions and involves the concept of sharing food with god(s). Food was used as an act of placation or a bargain with God for favors, or as a simple act of worship and gratitude. In the Biblical stories, Abraham slaughtered the lamb as a sacrifice. Cain brought the best of his produce and Abel the first born of his flock for their God. Roman and Greek mythology is rife with stories of sacrifices. The Aztecs made huge loaves, in the shape of Gods, which were thrown to the people to eat. The Hindus' worship includes offerings of produce or livestock that is thrown into the sacred fire with the chanting of mantras.

Food taboos abound in all cultures and religions.

> *"And the Lord God commanded the man, saying, Of every tree of the garden thou mayest freely eat:*
> *But of the tree of the knowledge of good and evil, thou shalt not eat of it."*
> —Genesis 2:16, 17: kjv

The disobedience in partaking of the forbidden fruit is said to have led to man's subsequent fall from grace. Jews and Arabs do not eat pork based on the Old Testament teachings.

> *"And the swine, because it divideth the hoof, yet cheweth not the cud, it is unclean unto you: ye shall not eat of their flesh."*
> —Deuteronomy 14:8 kjv

Hindus avoid beef, seeing the cow as a sacred animal that provides milk and labors in the field.

Buddha went through a period of experimentation with various forms of dietary restriction, including eating only a grain of rice a day, only to come to the realization that spiritual illumination and starvation or deprivation were not compatible. It was when he took care of his body that he realized enlightenment. Thus the Buddhist way is to look after the body and avoid extremes of overindulgence or abstinence.

A period of fasting is advocated in the major religions of the world. It is one of the five pillars of Islam. Fasting is thought to be a way to earn the approval of Allah, wipe out sins, and understand the suffering of the poor. There has been a recent resurgence in this country of fasting as a cleansing therapy. There have been no studies to show the health benefit of prolonged fasting. In fact, it may be dangerous in certain medical conditions such as diabetes with the risk of hypoglycemia, seizures or coma.

Neither has there been conclusive evidence for the so called detoxification diets and procedures. The body has multiple mechanisms for cleansing or detoxification when it is at optimal health. The respiratory system clears the body of nitrogen and carbon dioxide. Mucus production and the cough reflex helps to clear the passages of bacteria and foreign particles. The liver and gastrointestinal tract have multiple mechanisms of getting rid of toxins and waste products that are eliminated in the stool. The kidneys also have a dual function of selectively conserving important elements and eliminating waste. Being aware of this and taking time for the body's natural elimination functions is important to the overall general wellbeing.

Fad diets such as the "no carbohydrate", high fat and high protein diets have come and gone. These may work in the short term for the sole purpose of weight loss but rationally cannot sustain the needs of the body.

The basis of a healthy diet includes the three *macro* nutrients, which are protein, (found in fish, meat, poultry, dairy products and vegetables), carbohydrates (fruits, beans, pasta, rice and grains) and fat (found in meats and dairy products, nuts and oils). These three fundamentals provide the calories or fuel for the body to run on much like gas for the car.

Proteins are made up of amino acids that are vital for health. Foods from animal sources provide the essential eight amino acids which are essential for building, maintenance and repair of all tissues such as the skin, organs and muscle. They are also the components of the immunological and hormonal system. Vegetarians need to eat a large variety of foods to obtain the essential nutrients found in animal proteins.

Carbohydrates are the major source of glucose which provides the energy or fuel for cell function and physical activity. The healthiest sources of carbohydrates are whole grains, vegetables, fruits and beans. These also promote good health by providing vitamins, minerals and fiber. Fiber provides bulk to stools and assists in normal bowel function. Fiber is a prebiotic, which means it promotes the growth of good bacteria in the gut.

Fats are a concentrated form of fuel harboring more than twice the amount of fuel than carbohydrates and therefore an efficient way to store excess calories. When we eat more calories than we need, the excess is stored as fat. Fats are also essential for the absorption of certain vitamins and contribute to the structure of each cell. A layer of fat allows for padding of tissues and insulation against cold. Fats also add taste to foods. However animal fats and the hydrogenated fats, like the sticky grease on pans, tend to plug up arteries and increase the incidence of strokes and heart attacks. Vegetable oils on the other hand, like solvents that dissolve thick paints, do not stick to arteries and are heathier for the body.

The *micro* nutrients are the vitamins and minerals which are generally needed in small quantities to facilitate the chemical enzymatic reactions and functions of each cell. There are proven benefits to taking adequate amounts of calcium, magnesium and vitamin D for bone health. Excess calcium however, can upset the body's delicate balance and lead to calcium deposits and kidney stones.

In spite of unsubstantiated claims, supplements in the form of vitamins have become a multimillion dollar industry. Making healthy food choices generally would provide a large part of the body's need of these micronutrients. Note that these are micronutrients i.e. needed in small amounts for health and well-being. Exceeding the optimum level leads to toxic effects in the body. Mega vitamin supplementation is harmful and toxic to the body.

It is totally unnecessary and a waste of money.

Sixty-five percent of the human body is water. It is important to keep the body well hydrated. An adequate intake of fluids cannot be stressed enough. However the dangers of fluid overload needs to be kept in mind. Over-hydration can lead to fluid overload with resulting hyponatremia (low salt), edema (swelling) and elevated blood pressure. Thirst is not always an accurate indication of the body's need for water. The body's need for water fluctuates according to the environmental temperature, activity level and illness. On an average, forty-eight to sixty-four ounces a day is an adequate daily intake.

Although alcohol would be considered a fluid, it is high in calories and associated with far too many side effects. The cardiovascular benefits of alcohol have been touted by the industry (and also unfortunately by the medical profession) and more people are tending to take a drink or more on a daily basis. The risks of alcoholic cardiomyopathy, alcoholic encephalitis, gastritis, cirrhosis of the liver, testicular atrophy and mood instability are risks that have been minimized by the liquor industry. The threshold for irreversible damage from the toxic effect of alcohol, varies from individual to individual. The fetal alcohol syndrome is clear evidence that alcohol harms human tissues including the brain. Mood changes, aggressive behaviors, violence in the home, and road traffic accidents are also attributed to excessive alcohol intake.

The key essentials for healthy eating are to eat a variety of foods incorporating greens, colored vegetables, whole grains, fruits and meats. Eating regular meals with moderate portions to maintain a healthy weight is encouraged.

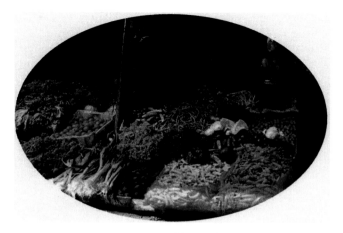

Vegetable stand, Sri Lanka

Medical Applications

Allergies and intolerances to foods abound in today's society. It is not always picked up with allergy testing. The common foods that create problems are nuts, seafood, strawberries, and oranges. Monosodium glutamate (MSG) which is added to foods as a flavor enhancer, can be a trigger for migraine headaches and gastrointestinal upsets. A large proportion of people, especially of African and Asian ethnic populations, are intolerant to milk and milk products. Milk is the natural food for baby. As we grow older, we lose the lactase enzyme necessary for processing the lactose sugar in milk; this leads to gaseous distension, abdominal cramps and diarrhea. Avoiding the offending foods is generally the best solution to prevent the ill-effects of allergies and intolerances.

Diabetes is a common affliction affecting significant proportion of the adult population and is becoming more prevalent in the younger age groups; with obesity and a less active lifestyle becoming the norm.

Sugar is an essential ingredient for normal functioning of every cell in the body. It is much like gas is for the functioning of a car. The car does not run without gas and the engine chokes up if the tank is overfilled. In a healthy young adult the average blood sugar runs between 80-120 mg /dl in the fasting state and 160 mg/dl two hours after meals. There may be an upregulation of these normal values as we age. Which is probably why overly aggressive treatment of blood sugars in the elderly lead to poor outcomes. Low blood sugar levels (hypoglycemia) and high blood sugars (hyperglycemia) are detrimental to the body. With diabetes, the hormone insulin is not adequately produced by the pancreas, or the way the body processes sugar becomes impaired. This is a simplistic model of diabetes. Many other factors influence blood sugars.

Blood sugar levels in diabetics tend to show wide fluctuations. The natural checks and balances involved in blood sugar equilibrium have gone awry. Excess sugar chokes multiple organs and vascular systems eventually leading to kidney failure, heart attack and stroke.

The goal in diabetics therefore is to keep the blood sugars in equilibrium as close to "normal" at all times, reducing excessive peaks and dips.

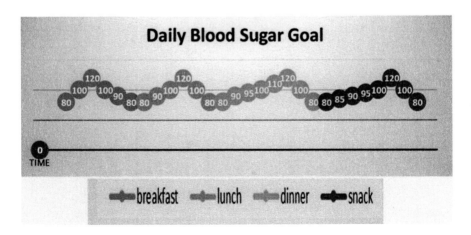

In diabetics, the blood sugar level peaks two hours after a meal (1 hr. in non-diabetics) then falls back to resting values. Different foods are metabolized at various rates in the body. This rate of metabolism is quantified numerically as the glycemic index (GI). Foods that cause a rapid rise in blood sugar are given higher values. Pure glucose is given a Glycemic Index (GI) of one hundred. A cup of sugar would cause an immediate spike of sugar, with a rapid drop often dipping below normal. Whole grains cause less of a spike and a more even level compared to simple carbohydrates. Fats being metabolized slowly have a longer life in the body with a much lower peak. Eyeing the chart below, we can appreciate that having a mix of complex carbohydrates, proteins and fats as well as having small frequent meals would result in more sustained, constant blood sugar levels.

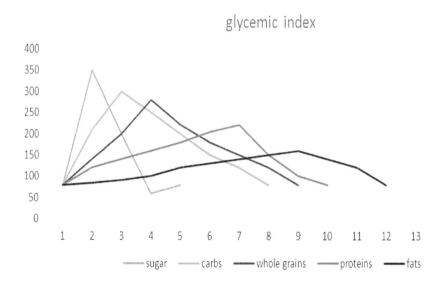

The next key to blood sugar control is frequent monitoring of blood sugars. It would be ideal to have a sensor that is applied to skin that displays blood sugar levels continuously. This technology is not available for general use as yet. So the option is for inter-mittent assessments using a home blood sugar monitoring kit.

By testing blood sugars before a meal and two hours after the same meal, we can infer that the difference in readings was the result of the meal consumed. A difference of more than 60 mg. flags the meal. Changes can be made in the portions and types of food in subsequent meals to maintain blood sugar goals. To min-imize the number tests a day the various mealtimes are tested at different days of the week.

Exercise burns off excess sugar and medications may be needed for optimum control of diabetes, but diet is the fundamental and cru-cial factor. As we will see in subsequent chapters, diabetes, hyper-tension and cholesterol are closely tied together with weight gain. Following the diet for diabetes will also lead to weight control as well as improvement in high blood pressure and cholesterol levels.

Meditative Exercise

Indulge in a culinary expedition and explore the flavors of the world. Visit a restaurant offering different ethnic foods. Try new recipes.

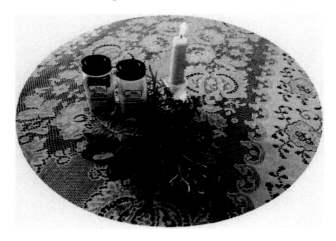

Experiment with the herbs and spices of the various cultures. Take time to experience the textures and tastes of foods. Thich Nhat Hanh describes the practice of mindfully savoring one raisin at a time.

Share a meal with friends and family. Using fresh produce, make a simple, nutritious meal paying attention to the balance of food groups. Prepare the meal with love and care infusing the meal with positive energy. The intimacy over food allows for lively conversation and connection. As the Irish proverb says, *"Laughter is brightest where food is best."*

Saying a blessing before each meal is a beautiful tradition to express gratitude for the abundance that the earth has to offer. Acknowledge the sacrifice of plant and animal that went into the preparation of your meal. As you gather around the table, extend the right hand to the one next to you with palms down in the giving position and accept the hand of the one to your left in the receiving position with the palms up. Life is about give and take. With mindfulness and gratitude partake of the meal and enjoy.

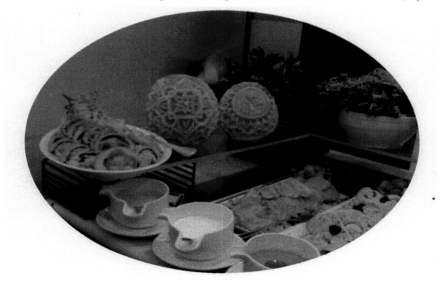

Chapter 5
EXERCISE

"The important thing in the Olympic Games is not to win, but to take part;
The important thing in life is not triumph, but the struggle;
The essential thing is not to have conquered but to have fought well."

—Coubertin

"Never trust a spiritual leader who cannot dance"
—Miyagi in "The Next Karate Kid"

In the stone ages, the lifestyle of hunting and gathering promoted a level of physical endurance. It was the survival of the physically fit as the hunter gatherers had to track game, skin the animals, fashion tools and build shelters as they were constantly on the move. The women folk also stayed physical—preparing, cleaning, cooking and looking after the children and the aged.

In Greek and Roman cultures, there were religious implications to being physically fit. The Olympic Games in 776 BCE were dedicated to the Greek God Zeus as the gods "championed" a winner. The Games aimed to show the physical qualities and accomplishments of young people. In Sparta, the belief that strong women would bear strong warriors prevailed, and women also were encouraged to be athletic. Warring communities, in order to protect their territories, trained men to be physically stronger to fight neighboring clans.

With industrialization and technological advancements, communities have become more sedentary. Our society has become increasingly inactive with the advent of cars, public transportation, escalators, remote controls and computers. As a result, sixty percent of adults in America are overweight, and obesity is becoming more prevalent even in children. An excess of body fat around the waist (central obesity), low HDL cholesterol and elevated blood sugar are the established factors for the metabolic syndrome. This syndrome is the precursor to the chronic conditions of hypertension and diabetes, increasing the risk of heart disease and stroke. With time as the disease progresses, complications and organ failure sets in followed by premature death.

Obesity is linked with an increase in plasma triglycerides and low density lipids, leading to fatty liver and gall bladder disease. One measure of obesity is the body mass index (BMI) which is calculated by dividing one's weight in kilograms by the square of one's height in meters. A value less than twenty-five is normal and more than forty is morbid obesity. Another measure is the abdominal circumference which is an even greater indicator of potential ill health. The current recommendation is to maintain abdominal girth of less than forty inches (102 cm.) in men and thirty-five inches (88 cm.) in women. These figures are merely guidelines based on a healthy young adult and one should not overly obsess about reaching these goals. The abdominal cavity is a potential space which can store large amounts of fat. This omental fat has been found to secrete multiple harmful chemicals such as leptin, adiponectin and inflammatory substances called cytokines. The hormone leptin that is over-produced in fat tissue leads to metabolic changes that promote further fat accumulation. Inflammatory cytokines raises C-reactive protein which increases production of super-oxides which damage tissues. Damage to the blood vessel lining or the endothelium is a precursor to heart attacks and strokes.

Exercise combats weight gain and reduces risk factors for cardiovascular disease. The American College of Medicine recommends thirty minutes of exercise, three to five times a week for health and longevity. What is probably more important is consistency in incorporating exercise into our weekly/daily routine. Participating in a physical activity that is pleasurable, interesting and stimulating contributes to staying on the program for a longer period of time. Any activity that is done mindfully to increase the range of movement and stimulate muscles and joints is beneficial. It is helpful to vary the activity to target bone and muscle strength, flexibility, stability and cardiovascular fitness. Walking, swimming, bicycling, gardening and dancing are all excellent forms of exercise.

Dance is integral in Egyptian and African lore. Dances were used to express joy and sorrow, to invoke prosperity and avoid disaster. The spirituality of dance is also seen in the whirling dervishes of the mystic Sufis, where the dancers reach spiritual heights with their dance. It is conceivable that the very first choreographers were the medicine men of primitive cultures. Their rhythmic dance evolved as a ritual to ask favors of their gods.

Agnes de Mille says that to dance is to be out of yourself—larger, more beautiful and more powerful. This inherent need to move rhythmically is seen in children who spontaneously express themselves in dance moves when exposed to music.

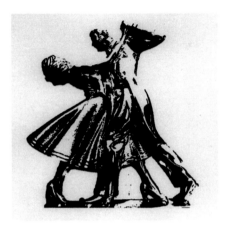

In contrast to the Western concept of physical exercise, the eastern view focuses on transformation and personal growth. The practice of yoga consists of a series of postures (asanas). It includes breathing and meditation and teaches patience in the face of difficulty. It requires an acute body awareness and focus. Similarly Tai Chi involves set patterns that flow into each other in a moving meditation. These exercise systems reduce stress, integrate mind and body, and cultivate inner, spiritual strength. They also increase balance and stability which are extremely helpful factors that minimize the risk for falls as we age.

One is never too old to start an exercise program. Studies have shown that even individuals in their eighties and nineties retained the ability to participate in an exercise program and reap its health benefits.

Whatever activity is chosen, it should be enjoyable and built up gradually. Doing it with another or a group usually boosts the pleasure derived and enhances social bonding. It is important to use common sense and exercise at one's own pace without pushing past exhaustion. Over-exerting, especially when tired, is when injuries and strains occur. Honor the body, and acknowledge its strengths and limitations.

Medical Applications

Strengthening and maintaining the flexibility of the back muscles reduces back pain eighty percent of the time. The bones and muscles act as an interconnecting support system for the physical body. The diaphragm is intrinsically related to the psoas muscle. Slouching and poor breathing habits causes a change in alignment of this relationship. A tight psoas muscle transmits this tension to the legs and feet resulting in aches and pains. Tension in the psoas muscle pulls the lower vertebrae forward causing slippage and narrowing of the nerve canals, ultimately compressing the nerves leading to sciatica.

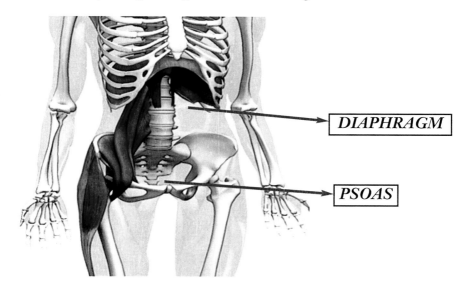

image adapted from wikimedia commons/bandhayoga.com
Author: Raymond Long, MD

Chronic back, neck and shoulder pain is often related to poor posture. With poor posture the muscles around a joint are imbalanced—one muscle group becomes stretched and weak and the opposing muscles become contracted and tight. For example, shoulders that are hunched cause tension in the pectoral or chest muscles, and stretched, weakened muscles between the shoulder blades at the back, resulting in upper back pain.

Physical fitness is linked inseparably to personal effectiveness in every field. Cognitive function and memory are improved. Studies show a decreased incidence of Alzheimer's in people who exercise. Exercise improves psychological well-being with less fatigue, anxiety and depression. It calms and clears the mind. The pleasure derived from exercise helps to stimulate natural serotonin which is a mood elevator. Sleep is deeper and more refreshing with regular exercise.

Cardiovascular function is improved with exercise. Exercise lowers blood pressure, strengthens the heart muscle, reduces body fat, increases the protective (good HDL) cholesterol and decreases the bad (LDL) cholesterol. Blood flow to all organs is improved. The improvement in lung function is especially helpful in asthmatics or people with compromised lung function. The immune system is strengthened making the body is less susceptible to illness.

Exercise is anti-aging as it reverses, to some degree, the changes seen in bone, joint and soft tissue. As we age our bodies tend to lose muscle mass, the muscles tend to shorten and the connective tissue or fascia (padding between muscles) becomes stiff. These changes lead to muscle imbalances and multiple aches and pains. This soft tissue rheumatism is classically seen in fibromyalgia.

Degenerative or arthritic changes occur in joints that aggravate disability, dysfunction and pain. Gentle range of motion exercise actively lubricates the joints and slows down the degenerative processes.

Osteoporosis or softening of the bones leads to the risk of multiple fractures. Collapse and shortening of the spinal bones or vertebrae results in the hunched posture and loss of height. Weight bearing exercises strengthens and molds the bones, delaying osteoporosis. Exercise has been more beneficial than any medication for bone health.

Bone density scores are based on a healthy young adult. It does not accurately represent bone strength in the aging population and should not be applied too aggressively in treatment decisions, especially since current medications for osteoporosis is often poorly tolerated.

Meditative Exercise

Lay on your back on a firm surface. Focus on gentle abdominal breathing as in chapter two. Visualize the breath and the heart's steady action pumping blood and oxygen to every muscle. Focus with the mind, be aware of each body part and experience the subtle changes that occurs with each breath.

Raise a leg from the hip as high as you can, without strain, keeping the knee extended. Flex and then rotate the ankle. Stretch a leg to one side opening out the pelvis and then to the other side crossing over the other leg in a scissor movement. Repeat each movement five to ten times and equalize the body by repeating the movements on the opposite leg.

Relax then flex both knees to the chest, return to neutral.

Lay on the right side of your body with knees bent. Stretch your arms forward in line with your shoulders. Raise your left arm up as you exhale allowing it to drop on your left as close to the floor as you can. Allow your head and gaze to follow its path, twisting at the waist. Your head faces away from the knees. This allows a stretch in the upper back as well as the pectoral muscles and achieves an opening of the chest wall. Take two deep breaths in this position before returning to neutral. Repeat on the opposite side.

In the standing position, focus on stacking the joints to improve posture—the neck over the shoulders, ribs over hips, and hips over heels. The pelvis and spine should be in neutral position.

Tuck the chin in, tuck the belly button towards the spine. Imagine the pelvis as a bowl. Tilt the pelvis forward and upward as if to prevent spill from the bowl. Let your movements come from the center of the belly or the core. Core body movements maximize strength. Breathe in from the pelvic floor to the diaphragm. Imagine everything above the navel to be light and stretched upwards, counteracting the natural forces of gravity that tend to compress the spine. Everything below the navel is grounded and stable.

Rotate the neck in a clockwise direction followed by a counterclockwise roll. Progress to rotate the shoulders, wrists, hips, knees and ankles in turn. Squeeze the shoulder blades together in front and then behind.

In the laying down position, return to gentle relaxed breathing. Appreciate the sense of being energized and vitalized in your body. Give thanks for each breath and celebrate each step you take towards health.

Make a commitment to perform these simple exercises to greet the new day for enhanced physical and mental health.

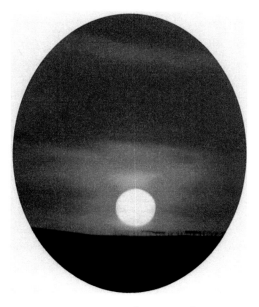

Sunrise, Singapore airport

CHAKRA 2

THE SACRAL CHAKRA
SIX PETALS OF THE SENSES

VISION   TOUCH

SMELL   TASTE

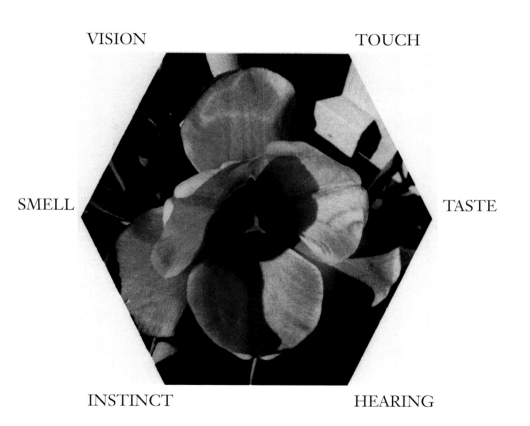

INSTINCT   HEARING

Chapter 6
SIX PETALS OF THE SENSES

"You must learn to heed your senses. Humans use but a tiny percentage of theirs. They barely look, they rarely listen, they never smell, and they think that they can only experience feelings through their skin."
—Michael Scott, The Alchemyst

Traditionally, the location of the second chakra is the sacral plexus. It is said to be located at the level of the sacrum above the coccyx. It is described to be "the seat of self." In other words this is how an organism perceives itself as separate from the environment. Single-cell life forms receive and process information from the outside environment, whether that information pertains to the availability of nutrients, changes in temperature, or variations in light. The cell's membrane interacts with the environment and responds to it by attraction or repulsion.

"The primitive self is realized at the interface between the inner biological processes of the human body and the external environment"
—Roy Baumeister

In this same context, human beings with their sense organs depend on interactions with the environment for their sense of self. (I am using self-hood here in its limited primitive sense and not in the modern psychological interpretations, which refers to the ego, learned behaviors, memory, emotions and social expectations.) We see this clearly in babies, as they focus with their eyes on the face of their mother, root towards the nipple and discover their mouths, hands and feet.

A sense is the faculty by which stimuli from the outside is perceived. Our senses connect us to the external world and are bridges between the outer world around us and our physical inner world. Through the five sense organs of the eyes, nose, tongue, ears and skin we perceive the five senses of sight, smell, taste, hearing and touch.

In Buddhist literature, the senses appear in allegorical representation as five horses drawing the "chariot" of the body, guided by the mind as chariot driver. Essentially the sense organs turn physical phenomena like light, sound, or pressure into electrical impulses. Bundles of nerve fibers carry these impulses to the brain to be interpreted. Sensations are brief unless further processed by the brain. Sensory data passes through the thalamus, and routes them to specific areas of the cortex— for example, the auditory cortex in the temporal lobe for hearing, the visual cortex in the occipital lobe for sight. The brain makes sense of these incoming sensory electrical signals, which puts this information in the context of memory, emotion, and cognition to perceive the whole picture.

To these five senses I would posit instinct as the sixth sense. Compare this with Daniel Siegal's interpretation of sixth sense as being the bodily signals or interoception. Instinct is the innate predisposition of a living organism towards a particular complex behavior that is not learned or based on prior experience. Sexual behavior and child rearing are seen as complex behavior with an instinctive basis.

Instinctively there is a need for preservation of the species with reproduction and replication. This function is tied in with sexual attraction, seeking out a mate as well as nurturing of the new born infant. This evolutionary, biological phenomenon of sexual lure is evident in birds and animals. The peacock shows off with its gorgeous, elaborate tail. The female elephant secretes a strong odor in her urine when seeking a mate. This sexual attraction is more than the appreciation of the five senses in that the attraction occurs specifically during the mating season. In humans, sexual desire seems to be greatest at the time of ovulation, although the existence of sex pheromones (chemicals secreted to impact the behavior of members of the same species) is not irrefutably proven.

The senses allow us the positive experience of hedonistic, sensuous pleasure. Pleasure and pain are the flip sides of the same coin. The same senses can lead to the perception of pain as a protective or aversive mechanism. The great philosopher Epicurus claims that some pleasures lead to great pains, and some pains are worth going through as they lead to greater pleasures.

The ultimate physical experience of pleasure is the sex act. Being in tune with one's senses allows one to key into one's ability to derive pleasure from life. By the same token, greater awareness of the body's senses enhances sexual pleasure.

"If we lose sight of pleasures and luxuries that intoxicate the senses in the most sensuous and beautiful and simplest of ways, then we've lost a lot"
—Savannah Page

Reward and pleasure typically serve to reinforce or motivate beneficial activities. Pleasurable activities can help to induce healthy behavioral changes and stimulate personal growth. However, as Epicurus states, *"By pleasure we mean the absence of pain in the body and of trouble in the soul. It is not by an unbroken succession of drinking bouts and of revelry, not by sexual lust, nor the enjoyment of fish, and other delicacies of a luxurious table, which produce a pleasant life; it is sober reasoning, searching out the grounds of every choice and avoidance, and banishing those beliefs through which the greatest tumults take possession of the soul."*

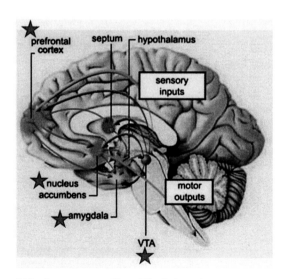

http://thebrain.mcgill.ca/flash/pop/pop
Taken from The Brain from Top to Bottom under copyleft

Engaging in simple daily pleasures using the senses can lead to stress reduction and an activation of the relaxation response. In the brain the pleasure circuit involves the neurons of the ventral tegmental area, the nucleus accumbens and prefrontal cortex. The amygdala enriches the experience with emotion, and the hippocampus stores it in memory.

Neurotransmitters such as dopamine, GABA, glutamate, serotonin, endorphins, cortisol and oxytocin are released in the experience of pleasure and euphoria. These chemicals possess calming and anxiolytic capacities, thereby facilitating feelings of well-being.

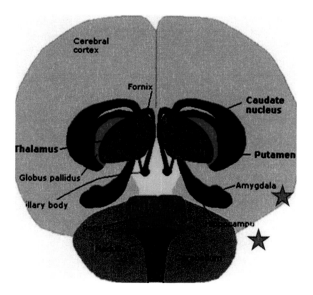

The brain splayed out and viewed from the undersurface. Adapted from Wikimedia commons. http://my-brainnotes.com/ subcortical-brain-diagram.gif

Too much dopamine however is toxic to the nerve cells. Therefore the brain controls and modulates the pleasure response by feedback mechanisms to metabolize and remove dopamine after the initial release. Pleasure seeking through recreational drugs stimulates the same system. However the intense stimulus from these drugs floods the synaptic space with dopamine so the feedback mechanism is insufficient to remove the excess. This leads to toxic effects in the brain including negative behaviors, addiction and diminished self-control.

Thus we see that the five senses, employed in sensing and appreciating the environment, and the sixth sense for propagation of the species are necessary for survival and can be pleasurable or sometimes painful or protective experiences. These are the six petals of the second chakra.

The second chakra is given the color of orange. Orange is a secondary color, a cross between red and yellow. The color orange radiates warmth and happiness or pleasure. Amongst artists it is the color of festivity and amusement. Orange is a naturally occurring pigment found in minerals, and foods such as apricots, mangoes, carrots, and saffron. It is said to be a color that is stimulating to the appetite. Many restaurants use pastel versions of orange, such as apricot or peach, or deeper versions such as terracotta, for their décor to increase the appetite and promote conversation and social interaction. It is the color of the robes of Buddhist monks and sadhus or holy men of India. It is the color of autumn when leaves turn color, signifying transformation.

The following chapters expand on the six senses of the second chakra.

Chapter 7
THE SENSES

"When you see an object, really look,
Hear sounds, Inhale scents,
Taste delicious flavors, Feel textures.
Use the objects of the five senses
and you will soon attain Buddhahood"
                          —Chakrasamvara Tantra

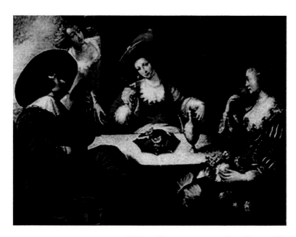

The five senses, by Jan Cossiers

VISION: The Faculty of Sight

In Greek mythology, Theia was revered as the goddess of sight and the shining light of the clear blue sky. She was the mother of three, Helios, god of the sun; Eos, goddess of the dawn; and Selene, goddess of the moon. Theia and her husband, Hyperion, allowed the world to be perceived by the light of their offspring. The Ancient Greeks believed that the eyes emitted a small beam of light that allowed them to see.

We now know that the human eye is an extremely complex organ. It acts much like a camera. Light passes through the pupil, is refracted by the lens and focused onto the retina which acts like a photographic film, processing the signals using dozens of different kinds of neurons. This is then converted into an electrical signal and relayed to the occipital lobe in the brain which translates it into images. The eyes and the nervous system do the sensing, the mind does the perceiving.

From the moment you wake up in the morning to the time you go to sleep at night, your eyes are acting like a video camera. Everything you look at is sent to your brain for processing and storage. What we see is data to allow us to know our bodies and the exterior world in which we live. The eye appreciates shape, color, movement, depth and distance.

The senses need stimulation during early "critical periods" of childhood development to form necessary neural connections. If an eye is covered for the first six months of life, it may remain functionally blind even after it is uncovered.

The esthetics of what is perceived varies from person to person and different cultures have varying standards of what is pleasing to the eye. This is easily appreciated in the art forms of different cultures. Japanese gardens are designed to simulate nature in attractive, balanced designs incorporating mountains (rocks) streams and waterfalls. The ancient Chinese system of Feng Shui, considers the placement of entry ways and furniture in an attractive display to promote Chi or wellbeing.

Visual perception isn't a passive receiving of inputs because we actively interpret, anticipate and pay attention to different elements of the visual world. As Henry David Thoreau so aptly says, *"The question is not what you look at but what you see."* We so often close our eyes to the beauty of nature all around us from the smallest wild flower to the brilliance of a setting sun in our busy, frenzied lives. We so often only see what we want to see. Helen Keller's answer to a comment that it must be hard to be blind was, that it would be, if she had no vision. The gift of sight goes beyond seeing. There is a Tlingit saying, *"There are two ways of seeing; mouse vision and eagle vision. The mouse only sees what is ahead of him. The eagle sees far into the future."*

Meditative Exercise

Spend a few minutes changing focus of your gaze from a distant object to a close object. Rotate the eyeballs to the four corners clockwise and counterclockwise. Rub your palms together vigorously to kindle warmth. Place the palms of the warmed hands over the eyes for a few seconds. Rub the palms again then use the index and middle fingers slightly spread apart to massage the upper and lower lids from side to side.

While driving to work gaze at the beauty around you—a cloud formation in the blue sky, a tree with spreading branches or the stark symmetry of modern architecture. We tend to miss the simple beauty all around us, preoccupied with our daily aggravations and bustling lives. Spend a day amongst nature or in a fine arts gallery. Cultivate the art of seeing with eyes that are open to deeply experience life and all its pleasures.

As you interact with clients or coworkers, look beyond the façade of the outer form into the person within. When you gaze into the eyes of a loved one see their history, their loves, joys, sorrows and the person he/she has become. Take time to connect with people for a richer, wholesome life.

HEARING—Perception of Sound

> *"The art of conversation is the art of hearing as well as of being heard."*
> —William Hazlitt, Selected Essays, 1778-1830

Fossils have allowed us a peek back in time to trace the development of complex body parts like the ear. Our reptilian ancestors sensed what was happening around them by feeling vibrations in the ground, through the jawbone. This rudimentary hearing apparatus has evolved to the complex middle and inner ear. The middle ear, fully separated from the jaw, is superior in receiving air-borne sound. The middle ear also explains why mammals, as a group, have the sharpest hearing on earth and the greatest diversity of listening styles. Bats and dolphins can detect sound waves at the ultrasonic end of the bandwidth, and elephants and humpbacked whales can hear at the other end of the spectrum capturing the long, low sound emitted by their peers for miles around. Interestingly enough, dolphins can hear fourteen times better than humans, and dogs hear a wider range of frequencies than humans. Sensitive hearing made it possible for early mammals to coexist with the dinosaurs and other predatory species. In humans, as well as animals, the faculty of hearing provides data from the environment.

Reviewing the apparatus of the human ear one can appreciate the complexity of this organ. Hearing depends on the presence of sound waves, which travel much more slowly than light waves. Sound vibrations are picked up by the external ear or pinna, transmitted through the delicate membrane of the ear drum and amplified by a series of three tiny bones called ossicles. It is then sent to the fluid in the cochlea in the inner ear. Inside the cochlea are receptors called cilia or hair cells that are embedded in the basilar membrane. Vibrations that reach the inner ear cause the fluid in the cochlea to move in waves. The wave's frequencies determine the pitch, the amplitude, the loudness and the timbre of the perceived sound. These waves make the hair cells move to trigger impulses in the connected nerve cells. These nerve cells, through the auditory nerve, send impulses from the ear to the brain. In the brain, the thalamus and the auditory cortex, which is in the temporal lobe of the cerebrum, process this information.

A particular form of sound is music. Music probably originated prior to language and is deeply ingrained and central to our being. An infant responds to the soothing croon of its mother. The toddler very naturally sways to the rhythm of music. In Greek mythology, the Greek God Orpheus is depicted as the greatest of all poets and musicians; Orpheus's music and singing could charm the birds, fish and wild beasts, coax the trees and rocks into dance, and divert the course of rivers. With his music and song he was also able to coax Hades, God of the Underworld, to return his wife who had received a fatal snake bite, signifying the power of music.

The images and thoughts that come to mind with a sound are dependent on multiple factors such as state of mind and prior associations. For example, the cock's crow in the early hours of the morning is distressing for a late riser but is music to the farmer and a signal to start the day. The sound of the laughter of children playing can be annoying to one who is wrapped in a mentally demanding task. But if one joins in the activities of the children that laughter can be pleasant and welcoming.

The sound of the wind blowing, the crash of waves on the shore and the chirp of birds are more than just audible sounds. They can elicit emotions, moods and feelings. The sense of hearing links us to the rest of humanity at an emotional level through speech and language. From the earliest sounds of a primitive call humans have developed language as a means of communication; from words to phrases, sentences and verbalization of complex abstract thought. The beauty of words is captured in great works of literature and poetry.

"Everything in the universe is within you… You are the universe in ecstatic motion." And *"Raise your words, not voice. It is rain that grows flowers, not thunder."*
—Jalaluddin Rumi

On the flip side, the most basic and powerful way to connect to another person is to listen. We so often only hear what we want to hear. To really connect with another, one has to develop the skill of truly listening.

"Only from the heart can you touch the sky."

—Rumi

Meditative Exercise

Appreciate the myriad sounds throughout the day. Listen to bird-song in the morning, crickets in the evening and feel it in the depths of your soul. Take a trip to the beach on a stormy night and listen to the rain and the sounds of a thunderstorm. Appreciate and soak in the emotions it evokes.

Settle in your most comfortable chair. Let yourself relax and be open to whatever thought comes naturally. Let your breathing be soft and comfortable. Play softly a piece of music with nature sounds. Immerse yourself in the piece of music excluding all extraneous thoughts. Imagine yourself on a trail with vistas of the snow-capped mountains in the distance on one side and calm, cool water on the other. Let the natural rhythm of the sounds of nature envelop and hold you.

Take time to be with a loved one and really listen paying attention to the words. Mirror back the words to understand the thoughts behind the words and to really connect deeply. Appreciating and developing this gift of listening and hearing brings an added dimension of pleasure and wholeness to life.

SMELL—A Pleasant Whiff

"At no other time (than autumn) does the earth let itself be inhaled in one smell, the ripe earth."
—Rainer Maria Rilke, *Letters on Cézanne*

A myth is told about Floria, the goddess of flowers. She owned millions of smells. One day as she was walking in the clouds, she fell and landed on earth. Here the flowers took care of her and built a rainbow ladder out of their leaves and petals and helped her back to heaven. As a reward Floria showered her scents on the flowers.

Plants and animals and some inorganic matter have odors, i.e. they give off chemical substances which is picked up by the receptors in the nasal passage. These cells then send signals along the olfactory nerve to the brain. At the brain, they are interpreted as those sweet smelling flowers or that moldy cheese.

Ants lay down an initial trail of chemicals, known as pheromones, as they return to the nest with food. This trail attracts and guides other ants. As long as the food source remains, the pheromone trail will be continuously renewed. In cats and dogs, hormones present in the urine, serve to mark their claimed territory. Mice can distinguish close relatives from more distantly related individuals on the basis of scent signals.

Smells have an extraordinary power to bring us pleasure. A remembered whiff of pipe tobacco, a particular perfume, or a long-forgotten scent can instantly conjure up scenes and emotions from the past. It readily lends itself to poetry and prose.

> *"You have thrown into this world the fragrance of musk and perfume…*
> *A hundred thousand murmurs have resulted from this scent.*
> *That was tossed into the earth and into the air."*
> —Rumi

One of these "murmurs" is seen in the verse below by Christopher Morley:

These are the odors I love well:
The smell of coffee freshly ground;
The fragrance of a fumy pipe;
The smell of apples newly ripe.

Meditative Exercise

Lean back in your comfortable chair... Start with gentle breathing as before. Close your eyes and relax into every part of your body. Let yourself take a trip down memory lane. Recall from your childhood the fresh, warm scents from the kitchen—perhaps that of fresh baked bread or pumpkin pie. Imagine the smells of your vacations as a child—the smell of the sea or the pine trees. Remember the fragrances of adulthood that brings a smile to your face—the smell of babies' skin after a bath. Imagine laying your head on the chest of a loved one and breathing in his/her smell. Bask in the pleasure that smells can bring.

TASTE—A Delectable Sense

"I have the simplest tastes. I am always satisfied with the best."

—Oscar Wilde

Insects have taste organs on their feet, antennae and mouthparts and have a highly developed sense of taste. Fish can taste with their fins and tails as well as their mouth. Taste is a sense that allowed testing the food consumed and was therefore a matter of survival. Generally, a bitter taste was an indication of poisonous inedible food. Taste and sense of smell are closely linked. That is why either a bad taste or foul odor can bring about nausea or vomiting. Smells of appetizing foods promote the production of saliva, making them literally mouthwatering and stimulates gastric juices in readiness for digestion.

Our tongue and the roof of our mouth are covered with almost ten thousand tiny taste buds. Saliva in the mouth helps break down food. These food particles, through the receptor cells located in the taste buds, send messages through sensory nerves to the brain where the different flavors are appreciated. The main taste sensations are that of sweet, salty, sour and bitter. The Greek philosopher Democritus said that when you chew on your food and it crumbles into little bits, those bits eventually break into four basic shapes of round, triangular, angular or spherical to correspond with the four basic tastes. An interesting outdated theory totally disproved by science.

When taste buds were discovered in the nineteenth century, Kikunae Ikeda was at same time enjoying a bowl of dashi, a classic Japanese soup made from seaweed. He sensed that he was tasting something beyond the four well known taste categories. Ikeda went into his lab and found the secret ingredient. He wrote in a journal for the Chemical Society of Tokyo that it was glutamic acid. Glutamate is found in most living things, but when this organic matter breaks down with cooking or aging processes the glutamate molecule breaks down to give a delicious taste. And since then two new tastes were added to the classification: savory and pungent.

Imagine not being able to taste the different flavors of foods. A good part of life's simple pleasures will be lost.

Meditative Exercise

Bring taste to a higher level by participating in a wine and cheese tasting event. Experience the burst of pleasure with your first bite of a ripe peach or a chocolate covered strawberry. Be adventurous—take a trip to a foreign country, if able, or to a restaurant that serves cuisine from a different culture and taste foods that are strange to you. Enjoy these new gustatory explorations whether alone or with friends and family. Savor foods with intent and deliberation taking one bite at a time. See how that brings a new dimension of pleasure into your life.

TOUCH—A Healing Sensation

> *"Touch has a memory. O say, love, say,*
> *What can I do to kill it and be free?"*
>
> —John Keats

The layer of your skin called the dermis is filled with tiny nerve endings which sense the environment with which your body comes in contact. When touch, pain or heat sensors in your skin are stimulated, they send electrical pulses to your neurons or nerve cells. These sensory neurons pass the information to the spinal cord, which sends messages to the brain where the sensation is registered.

Research has shown how touch in the form of skin-to-skin contact between baby and parent is important for baby's development. They cry less and it helps them sleep better. Mothers embracing this close contact, are generally more relaxed and happy and more sensitive to their baby's cues. The relationship between parent and baby is enhanced with touch. We need to be held and to hold, to be touched and to touch. Nothing eases suffering like human touch. Physical touch makes us healthier; it reduces stress and boosts the immune system both for the one who offers it as well as the receiver.

A firm handshake with a friend can create a connection. As in the words of a popular song, by reaching out to touch somebody's hand we make the world a better place. Hands laid on shoulders in a gesture of comfort speaks louder than words. A hug from someone we care about can lower blood pressure and make us feel valued and important. Having a pet to cuddle and stroke helps to assuage loneliness. Since ancient times the gentle pressure from a massage or a warm spa experience has been known to be therapeutic.

Meditative Exercise

Take a walk in the park or the beach and feel the pleasure of the wind blowing on your face or the sand between your toes. Hug a tree and feel the surface of the bark. Compare the textures of different leaves in the park. Wear fabrics and use bedsheets that feel sensual to the touch. Feel the warmth of a child's spontaneous hug. Reach out to touch family and friends during a conversation where appropriate and see how that affects you as well as the reciprocal feeling it evokes in the other. Be aware that inappropriate touch can lead to mental anguish and suffering.

Take time out in your busy lives to experience an occasional day at a spa. As you move through the day, seek out opportunities to linger and appreciate the different sensations of touch.

Medical Applications

Pleasure is a peculiar sensation effected by nerve pathways. Pain and pleasure are generally perceived through neural pathways and interpreted in the higher centers of the brain. The same pathways of pleasure can generate pain. The brain produces neurotransmitters that generate pleasure but it can also produce neurotransmitters that generates pain. Topical rubs such as capsaicin, salon pas, or mentholatum, use this principle as a mechanism to counter pain.

The eyes with which one sees beauty can also see visions of pain and horror. War veterans after being subject to horrific scenes of death and carnage endure deep emotional pain. War veterans have high rates of post-traumatic stress disorders. We can extrapolate that horror movies and violence on TV shows can similarly affect the neural pathways to cause prolonged emotional pain.

Loud sounds from boom boxes, loud concerts, and noisy work environment can damage the delicate hearing organ and lead to impaired hearing. Using protective gear and toning down exposure to loud noises is suggested to reduce noise associated deafness. Excess wax build up in the ear canal can cause loss of hearing. A few drops of baby oil or mineral oil can soften wax to allow it to drain naturally. During the Greco-Roman times, honey, vinegar and cucumber juice was used to remove ear wax, although it is not a current recommended therapy. Tinnitus is another common affliction of the ear. It can be related to the natural aging process, or use of drugs such as aspirin or certain cancer medications.

Smell perception can be reduced or altered by allergies. Unpleasant smells can be a turnoff. Some genetic conditions are associated with an inability to smell. Medications, smoking, vitamin deficiencies, head injury, cancers, chemical exposure, and the effects of radiation can cause taste and smell disorders.

Flavor enhancers such as monosodium glutamate have been shown to be a trigger for migraine headaches. Food additives such as sulfur dioxide and nitric acid and preservatives have been linked with cancer, digestive problems, neurological conditions, ADHD, heart disease, and obesity. Sodium nitrite is added to meats to enhance and maintain an appealing and fresh red color. Sodium nitrite can produce cancer causing chemicals such as nitrosamines. Numerous studies have shown a link between cancer in humans that consume excess nitrite containing processed and cured meats. There is some evidence that a mix of additives commonly found in children's foods increases the mean level of hyperactivity.

Drug users seek heightened pleasure with drugs such as narcotics and hallucinogens which enhance sensations to cause a high by stimulating the pleasure centers and releasing dopamine and other neurotransmitters. However with the use of drugs, the neurons that release the dopamine become depleted and a vicious cycle of craving and need for more drugs develops. The continued use of drugs causes degeneration of the neurotransmitters initially causing drug tolerance and addiction and eventually to *personality changes and disorders*. Pleasure turns to pain and disease.

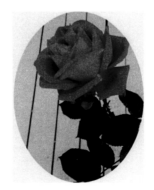

Chapter 8
INSTINCT

"The very essence of instinct is that it's followed independently of reason."

—Charles Darwin

"The natural man has only two primal passions, to get and beget."

—William Osler

Instinct and intuition often are used interchangeably. This is due to the limitation and inadequacy of language and our confusion of the precise nature of either term. Researching the definitions of these two terms:

Instinct: an innate, typically fixed pattern of behavior in animals in response to certain stimuli. Any behavior is instinctive if it is performed without being based upon prior experience or learning as an expression of innate biological factors.

Intuition: the ability to understand something immediately, (or a thing that one knows or considers likely from instinctive feeling) without the need for conscious reasoning.

For my purpose, the sixth sense is instinct, the special innate quality of knowing leading to a fixed pattern of behavior for the species. Instinct is essentially intrinsic and biologically based. According to the instinct theory of motivation, all organisms are born with innate biological tendencies that help them survive. Instinct is comparable to Sigmund Freud's *"id"*. The id is the part of the personality structure that contains a human's basic, instinctual drives. It is the source of our bodily needs, wants, desires present from birth. The id knows no value judgments: no good and evil, no morality. The mind of a newborn child is regarded as completely "id-focused," or instinct driven to demand immediate satisfaction of its needs.

Instincts are goal-directed patterns of behavior that are not the result of learning or experience. The goal is generally the preservation of the species. Motivation for this behavior is the feeling of pleasure inherent in the reward system of the brain.

The maternal instinct is to nurture and care for the young one. A mother's instinct is an inbuilt mechanism that enables a mother to protect, love and raise her child and keep it safe. In nature, mammalian mothers who were attentive and caring to their young were more likely to rear successful offspring. Brain scans suggest that particular circuits in the brain are activated to allow a mother to distinguish the smiles and cries of her own baby from those of other infants. The fact that a woman responds more strongly to her child's crying, than to its smiling, seems to be a biological adaptation associated with effective infant care.

In *Sex in the Wild* series on National television, an episode featured the birth of a baby kangaroo which weighed one pound.

The joey crawls up its mother's abdomen to land in the kangaroo pouch where it nurses and grows for six months before it finally leaves the pouch and fends for itself. Prior to this the mother kangaroo spends the last few days of its one-month pregnancy preparing the pouch by cleaning and licking off the scales to ensure that the pouch is soft and ready for joey. These behaviors of both baby and mother are not learned or copied.

The animal and insect kingdom is rife with instances that clearly show examples of the inborn patterns of behavior. Birds have an inborn nesting instinct in spring and migratory behavior in winter. Sea turtles newly hatched on a beach, will spontaneously move toward the ocean. The elaborate hierarchical social behavior of bees are further examples. Bees have a natural intelligence to care for the queen bee. The queen bee serves the purpose of laying eggs and perpetuating the species. The worker bees play a supportive role and by instinct lay wax and then excavate it in order to form cell after cell to form the architecturally amazing hexagonal bee hive to house the eggs and subsequently the larvae. Honey bees perform an elaborate dance to communicate the presence of a food source.

Psychologist Abraham Maslow argues that humans no longer have instincts because we have the ability to override them in certain situations. Instincts become more complex and almost unrecognizable with the cerebralization of man coupled with the complex phenomenon of socialization.

People are able to modify an action by becoming consciously aware of and altering their behavior. Animals, without a sufficiently strong volitional capacity, may not be able to change their fixed action patterns, once activated. However understanding the root of instinctual behavior is a step toward the understanding of human behavior. Nature builds on what was there rather than reinventing the wheel. As Ralph Waldo Emerson states, *"All progress is an unfolding, like the vegetable bud, you first have an instinct, then an opinion, then a knowledge, as a plant has root, bud and fruit."*

Mating and nesting rituals are further examples of instinctually motivated behavior in animals. Animals do not learn to do this, it is an inborn pattern of behavior geared toward successful survival of the species. Instinctively, women flaunt their femininity and enhance their physical beauty with a host of cosmetic products and adorn themselves with attractive clothing and jewelry to entice a man. Similarly men build up their muscles and assume macho behaviors to attract the softer sex. Just watch behaviors in a singles group!

It has been shown that many animals possess a vomeronasal organ (VNO) at the base of the nasal passage. The VNO is used to detect pheromones, chemical messengers that carry information between individuals of the same species. Its presence in many animals has been widely studied and the importance of the vomeronasal system to the role of reproduction and social behavior has been shown in many studies. A female elephant in heat releases chemical signals (pheromones) in her urine and vaginal secretions to signal her readiness to mate. A bull elephant will follow a potential mate and assess her condition by collecting these chemical signals with his trunk and sensing it with his vomeronasal organ.

The VNO sends neuronal signals to the accessory olfactory bulb and then to the amygdala, and ultimately hypothalamus which is part of the limbic system.

The amygdala and limbic system is known to be part of the "reward system" or the pleasure centers of the brain (see illus. pg. 52). Since the hypothalamus is a major neuroendocrine center affecting aspects of reproductive physiology and behavior (as well as other functions) it may explain how scents influence mating behavior. So we see that the vomeronasal organ connects to the amygdala of the brain and relays information about the surroundings in essentially the same manner as any other sense.

In humans the discovery of the cranial nerve zero or "terminal nerve" suggests that this nerve could be a vestigial nerve related to the sensing of pheromones as in animals. This hypothesis is further supported by the fact that the terminal nerve projects to the areas of the brain which are involved in regulating sexual behavior in mammals. Thus although the presence of the VNO and functionality in humans is debated, we can draw a parallel as to the evolutionary connection between the senses, sex and pleasure. Evolutionary concepts also help us understand the inherent power of the sex urge.

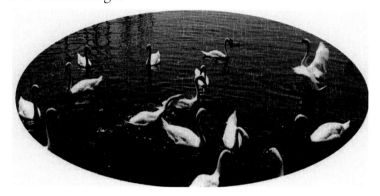

Swans, Lake Geneva

Chapter 9
LIFE

"Your children are not your children.
They are the sons and daughters of Life's longing for itself"
—Kahlil Gibran, *The Prophet*

"Life is a sexually transmitted disease"
—R.D. Laing

The fetus started as a single cell formed though the fusion of the ova and the sperm. The single cell divides and goes through processes that are not completely understood to form cells that are marked to become specific organs and structures. Soon a child that can eat, see, hear, run, and play materializes and before too long it becomes a young adult. How truly amazing that a single cell within a womb—the product of a sexual union, grows into a miraculous human being.

It is just as mind boggling how our universe has come into being. We see similar patterns being repeated over and over again in nature. This perception has been expounded by Benoit Mandelbrot in his conception of Fractals. Fractals are similar geometric patterns in nature; for example, a fern repeats the whole leaf pattern in its fronds. Fractals are not limited to geometric patterns but can also describe processes in time.

So the pattern of a single cell developing into a complex human being is a repetition of all life in its creation starting with a single cell and replicating to form complex organisms such as trees and animals and humans. The simplest single celled organism has unheard of complexity; this complexity exponentially increases up the evolutionary scale. Genetically, plant life has been shown to share many of the same genes as humans.

Life began with the first cell and has never been recreated since. We do not own life and neither can we force life to continue on ad infinitum. *"In the beginning was the word,"* (John 1:1 kjv)—or concept or idea; a mysterious energy blast that led to life. The sperm and the ovum are the carriers of life just like the torch bearer or a lamplighter passes on the flame or light. Life is not created with conception, but the potential for a human being (or animal) occurs with conception. With conception the new cell has the potential to grow and form a living organism that can ultimately survive on its own. The seeds of life continue to be passed on from generation to generation. Life expresses itself through us.

So what is life? The dictionary defines life as the condition which distinguishes the active organism from inorganic matter encompassing the capacity for growth and functional activity with self-sustaining properties. Often times when one walks into a room, one can be aware of a presence before seeing the person. There is that special something that emanates from a live individual that is vibrant and alive. This is the difference between life and death. I have been impressed on many occasions in the course of my work by the difference in aura, or rather lack of aura surrounding someone who has passed on. A person/animal who has

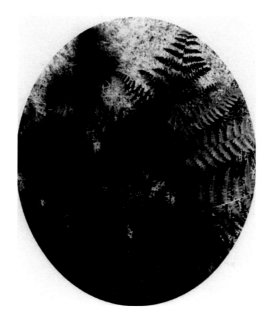

died has all the cells/chemicals and organ systems intact and in place. But yet there is no growth or functional activity, and is not self-sustaining. That life principle, the soul or whatever you conceive it to be, (distinct from all physical and chemical factors) is no longer there. Life is the energy through which we exist. It is with us till we die. Whether we believe in God or not, life is an undeniable fact. It is not essential to have belief systems to experience life. It is the energy that turns matter into form. It is the common principle linking all living things.

Sperm and ova are life forms as defined by the dictionary as it manifests growth and functional activity. They carry the potential for new life. The sperm and ovum are equally important in the process of reproduction. Both male and female share equally in the process of procreation.

Historically and currently, controversy exists about the moment of life ranging from the time of conception to the time of birth. The Jewish position had been that life occurred at the time of birth, equating breath with human life. They also believed that the mother's life took priority over the fetus. Pope Gregory the fourteenth declared that the "soul" entered the body at the time of quickening (the moment that fetal movements are felt) which he set at 116 days or sixteen weeks of pregnancy. Pope Pius, in 1869, changed that thinking and declared that "ensoulment" occurred at the time of conception. This change in thinking has led to the divisive and emotionally charged controversy around the issue of abortion.

Medically, for practical considerations we have arbitrarily determined life to be when the fetus is viable. With medical advances viability of the fetus has improved from thirty-two weeks in the 1960s to the current twenty weeks or when the fetus is 500 gm. A fetus is defined as the organism that is developing in the maternal womb eleven weeks after conception when body parts are formed. The first eleven weeks is known as the embryonic stage.

Historically, in early and primitive cultures, abortions were induced non-surgically using herbs such as pennyroyal and tansy. Some of the herbs used were toxic or poisonous and lead to maternal mortality. Physical means such as tight girdles, strenuous jumping up and down and punching of the stomach were also utilized. In the second century surgical instruments were introduced and used in procedures similar to modern-day dilation and evacuation. Maternal mortality was high as there was little knowledge of sterile procedures.

It was during the Victorian era, with Pope Pius' declaration, that abortion was made illegal, quoting the value of human life as a priori. This caused women to risk their lives seeking dangerous, illegal abortions underground from backstreet untrained personnel. To prevent death and disease associated with these underground procedures the pendulum swung back. Abortion became an accepted procedure under hygienic, safer conditions, flushing out the charlatans and improving conditions for patients. Over time stricter regulations were imposed on clinics, providers and clients seeking abortion which increasingly restricted access, especially for the poor.

These rules and laws pertaining to women's health issues, have been set by men in roles of power either religious or legislative. Men have divorced themselves from their role in the process of the formation of that new life. Feminists hold the position that *abortion is an undesirable necessity brought about by thoughtless men and that the perpetrator drove her to the desperate need for the procedure.* In our current society, the woman is made to live with guilt, anxiety, blame and shame if she makes a decision to abort a pregnancy (a potential life form) no matter what her unique situation is.

Men are bearers of the seed of life as much as women. Consider that with each ejaculation, millions of sperms (packages of potential life forms) are wasted or "killed." Genesis 38:9 Onan "spilled his seed" on the ground and was punished by death.

No matter what one's position is on the abortion issue we have to admit it is not black and white; multiple factors need to be considered on an individual basis. Pregnancy is not uncommonly the result of a man's forcible unwanted action on a woman in the form of rape. The woman has to bear the scars of that violation on her body and spirit for the rest of her life. The environment of maternal hostility and revulsion has a negative impact on the developing fetus. The single mother has the burden to care and provide for her child as the perpetrator would be long gone. The developing fetus and subsequently the child is a constant reminder of that trauma.

Medical Applications

A single fertilized egg divides to form a group of cells that can transform into all the structures of the human body. Early cells (stem cells) retain their ability to differentiate into different kinds of tissue cells when the need arises to repair damaged organs. Research into the basic mechanisms of cell development and differentiation, has offered the hope for new treatments for spinal cord injuries, type 1 diabetes, Parkinson's disease, Alzheimer's disease, heart disease, stroke, burns, cancer, and osteoarthritis using stem cells. New treatments and procedures invariably face judgement and controversy. We saw this with organ transplantation and in vitro fertilization, for example, which has proved to be life enhancing for many. We can keep our minds open to the far reaching benefits of these new advancements using stem cells.

Mindful Meditation

We can, with a change in perspective, look with compassion and tolerance on the woman who has to make that gut-wrenching decision to terminate her pregnancy, rather than spew hate and perpetuate violence. The death of compassion and genuine caring for another is the greater loss in life.

Take personal responsibility for one's own sexual behavior. Enter each sexual encounter in a more mindful way. Recognize that the male sexual organ is a "weapon of mass destruction" in that millions of sperms are wasted (killed) with each ejaculation. By the same token an egg is "wasted" each month before one is eventually fertilized. Loss and survival is part of nature's way.

Find a spot in a lovely, quiet garden. Abundant life surrounds you; the varied, succulent plants and birds with their happy song.

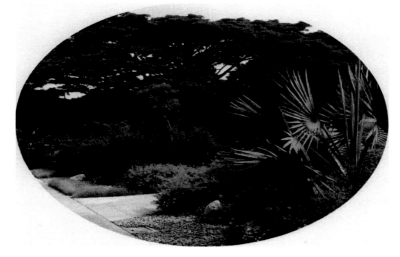

Hort Park, Singapore

Start with the breath as before to clear the mind. Contemplate on life and its origin whatever your beliefs may be. Envision the lives of generations that have gone on before. Give thanks for the lives of people you know and come in contact with.

Feel gratitude for the priceless gift of your own precious life.

Feel the wonder of your body and its incredible potential to bring forth new life. Reflect on the many gifts you have birthed.

Chapter 10
SEXUALITY

"What food is to a man's well-being, such is sexual intercourse to the welfare of the whole human race."
—Augustine

Sexual energy permeates all cultures and myths and the whole of human existence. We see it in the ancient drawings of the Egyptian tombs, the statues of India and the billboards in America. Confucius says, "Food and sex are natural urges." Lovemaking, or the "Art of Chambers" was not only an integral part of early Taoist spiritual teaching or meditation, it was also believed to be an important means to longevity. The Taoists advocate a total experience in sexual intercourse utilizing loving eye contact, caressing and touching. They believe that when two persons are in ultimate physical and emotional harmony, there is an exchange of yin/yang essences and a renewing of life's *vital* energy. According to Taoists, neither the man nor the woman should strive for fulfillment alone but consider each other's climax. The male is encouraged to prolong his own climax and to elevate his partner to a higher plateau of pleasure, and strive towards a simultaneous orgasm called "bursting of the clouds."

Freud perceived sexuality as a base instinct welling up from the unconscious and that humans are biologically inclined to seek sexual gratification. From an evolutionary standpoint, motivators in the brain have evolved to give us pleasure when we engage in sexual behavior as the incentive or reward to perpetuate the species.

The primitive brain or the limbic system plays a key role in sexual function in both humans and animals. The two major centers in the reward circuit, the ventral tegmental area (VTA) and nucleus accumbens receive sensory input (such as sight, smell, touch, etc.) from the amygdala. All of these centers are interconnected and innervate the hypothalamus. The hypothalamus then acts on the autonomic and endocrine functions of the entire body. The hypothalamus together with the pituitary gland releases neurotransmitters and hormones that orchestrate the necessary physiological needs of the body such as changes in heart rate, blood pressure and vasodilation that occurs with sexual excitement. In humans, unlike in animal species, the prefrontal cortex has the executive control and chooses whether to seek the reward.

Many cultures view sexual prowess as a symbol of one's maleness giving rise to the concept of "the Macho man." Giving in to primitive brain is not indicative of strength—true greatness lies in becoming master of the primitive brain and subjugating desires of the flesh. Aristippus of Cyrene (435 to 366 B.C.), the founder of the Cyrenaic school of philosophy, cautions "to exercise good judgment, to temper human passions."

Each major religion has established moral codes covering issues of sexuality, morality, ethics etc., which have sought to guide

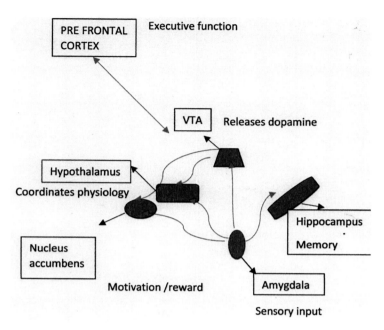

Mid Brain (limbic system)

people's sexual activities and practices. The Jewish faith emphasizes that sexual desire should be controlled and channeled only to be satisfied at the proper time, place, and manner, between husband and wife, out of mutual love and desire for one another. The Hindu precepts advocate training the mind before partaking of pleasure. Buddhists believe that attachment or fixation to desire, including sexual desire, leads to suffering.

During the Middle Ages, marriage came to be seen as a sacrament and therefore under the regulatory power of the Church. Throughout the middle ages, the Church was in constant battle with the open sexuality which prevailed from pre-Christian times. The primary purpose of sex according to the Catholic Church (and some other cultures) is to reinforce the marital bond and to procreate. The Catholic tenet was that sex was a gift from God and sex without reproduction was an abomination. In the eighth century, the Church tried to establish monogamous marriages as indissoluble, and popularized celibacy as the ultimate noble sacrifice.

The environment, culture, religion and social setting have played major roles in the evolution of perception, attitudes, and behaviors of sexuality. In ancient cultures, it was vital to have many offspring to help in looking after the property and the myriad chores in agricultural or farming communities. Women were therefore revered as the bearers of children. The wealthier you were, the greater the number of wives you had. Even to this day, we see this amongst some business men and the Mormon communities. With the advent of industrialization and the rise of cost of living, more and more couples are choosing to have two or no children. With reproduction being less of an imperative, society places pleasure as the definitive in sexuality. Sexual relationships, however, can lead to considerable emotional conflicts. It is not unusual that some, turned off by the emotional complexities of sexual entanglements, substitute and find pleasure in friendships and community rather than sexual relationships.

The emotional aspect of sexuality is pervasive throughout life. The infant expresses this through cuddling, suckling and the displeasure of wet diapers. The toddler engages in genital play. With puberty, body and related emotional awareness emerges. From then on sexuality deals with one's feelings about self and others. It is expressive of the desire for human closeness and intimacy and physical pleasure. Values and mental attitudes, with a clear understanding of expectations of the other, determine fidelity, commitment and the purpose of sexual expression.

When we look around us at nature we see a plethora of reproductive processes. We see asexual binary fission in the single-celled organism. Flowers use a 'middle man' or third party with bees; when bees visit flowers they brush against the pistil collecting pollen which is deposited on another flower to fertilize it. The reward for the bee is the nectar from the flowers. Earthworms are hermaphrodites having both male and female organs as part of its anatomy. A mating pair overlap ends and exchange sperm with the other. Dolphins and some other mammals although heterosexual, have been seen to engage in same sex encounters.

Homosexual and bisexual behavior is replete in Greek history. Sexual passion between men in Greece was considered normal, and often a mature male took a teen-aged youth to mentor. The Native American "two spirit" belief is that some people are born with the spirits of both genders. Native Americans place no moral judgment to love or sexuality; a person was judged for their contributions to their tribe and for their character. Two Spirit people were highly revered as people able to see the world through the eyes of both genders at the same time. Thailand and Indonesia also honor the spectrum of gender without stigma, recognizing five genders in their society.

Sex in humans is as varied as in nature. It is in the nature of things. One's sexual behavior and how we define ourselves and our relationship to others is a complex process involving multiple facets of life including family values, cultural norms, education and experience. One step toward wellness in this area is to question our own belief systems. Wellness is becoming comfortable in one's own skin and how we relate to others and their sexual values/behaviors. Accepting the way of others, honestly and without judgment, leads to maturity, self-understanding and tolerance.

One's sexuality is an integrated, individualized expression of one's unique self. It involves a sense of happiness with the way we are irrespective of our sexual orientation whether it is expressed or not. It involves self-acceptance and understanding of sexual behavior as an integrated whole.

Sex can be communication that is fun and pleasurable, serious or playful whether expressed with another or with self. Sex is part of life's purpose, but an undue preoccupation with sex diminishes one and detracts from all that life has to offer. With the sexual revolution of our times comes greater freedom of choice and the right to say when, where, how and with whom or to be sexually abstinent without judgment. It involves the absolute right to say "no" and be heard, honored, and respected. Our sexuality belongs to us. Choosing to engage in or abstain from sexual activity is a personal choice and never, ever to be forced on another.

Medical Applications

Sexually transmitted diseases are preventable for the most part with barrier contraceptives and pre-sex testing. Education and the availability of contraception has helped to decrease the incidence of teen and unplanned pregnancies.

It takes emotional maturity to acknowledge and assume the burden of responsibility for the consequences of sex. Pre-marital or couples counselling is a helpful tool to prepare one for the myriad aspects of relationship.

The dark side of sexuality emerges as rape, incest, pornography and prostitution. In these circumstances sex is a horrifying experience for the victim. Victims of rape and incest go through life with severe emotional problems. Giving in to the sexual instinct does not prove manliness as all animals and lesser organisms do it. With the higher cortical centers, an evolved human being brings awareness to exercise consideration, caution and control. This is the mark of a true man or woman.

Meditative Exercise

Ensure that you are well rested and have had a satisfying meal. Keep the room simply furnished and visually pleasing and at a comfortable temperature. Set the stage with soft music. Share a warm bath or shower and feel the closeness of your partner. Feeling fresh and clean prepare for a sensual massage. Using massage oils appreciate the sensation of touch and smell.

Massages are generally given in the bottom-to-top direction to counter forces of gravity, and blood flow. Be gentle and loving and deliver the strokes with intent. The skin, being the largest sex organ, has its own erogenous zones; so, allow yourself to discover these areas each time you give or receive massage. The most sensitive areas of the body are the hands, lips, face, neck, tongue, fingertips and feet. Aim on a balance between giving and receiving.

Focus on being heart centered, feeling positive emotions for your partner. Leave all distracting thoughts behind. Whatever your sexual orientation, bring wholeness to the experience. As you give from the heart also tune in to what your heart desires to receive in return.

Let every moment be a total consciousness of two people loving each other without striving for orgasm. As you harmonize your bodies experience a truly cosmic experience, or to put it bluntly the "big bang."

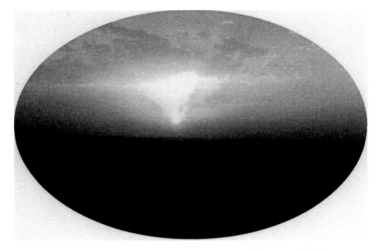

Sunrise, sand dunes of Morocco

Chapter 11
GENDER

"What greater thing is there for two human souls than to feel that they are joined for life—to strengthen each other in all labor, to rest on each other in all sorrow, to minister to each other in all pain, to be one with each other in silent, unspeakable memories at the moment of the last parting"

—George Elliott

Society is changing. The feminist movement has encouraged women to reclaim autonomy and their rightful place in the family and society. Women are participating in the work force and can no longer be expected to assume sole responsibility of the care of home and children. It is no longer necessary for women to deny their innate abilities, downplay themselves or play second fiddle to their husbands. Women are assuming roles as leaders and innovators. The feminine qualities of patience, tenderness and nurturing, so long discounted by men, are increasingly gaining attention and credibility in the work place. It is inevitable therefore that the old model of the family unit with male authority and female subservience can no longer be relevant. Adaptation and adjustments have to happen.

Evolution theories, promoted by Darwin, of environmental adaptation and change have been the scientific basis of the creation of new species.

Changes over millennium with breeding and interbreeding facilitated the evolution of our species: the Homo sapiens. Adaptive genetic changes are transmitted to the offspring, and ultimately these changes become common throughout a population affecting both males and females. We can see this clearly amongst African Americans who show marked changes in physical and behavioral characteristics as compared to the native African. Children adopted into another culture show different characteristics from their natural heritage.

Darwin's theories, however, do not explain the origin of the complex process of sexual reproduction and the differentiation of male and female or the evolutionary benefit of sexual reproduction. Male/female differentiation happened long before the human race. Nonetheless it is far-fetched to conceive the development of one sex to become 'the first male' without a parallel development in the formation of first female to allow sexual union.

We can therefore, appreciate that male and female evolved at the same time.

This perspective contrasts sharply with the Abrahamic traditions which describe the formation of first man, Adam, from mud or clay. First woman, so the story goes, was formed from the rib of Adam. Incidentally, the ancient Greek myths tell of the birth of Dionysus from the thigh of the Greek god Zeus. Woman was therefore viewed as an appendage, fostering the position of the supremacy of man. This view, unfortunately, was perpetuated by the apostle Paul in the New Testament with his outlook on sex and the inferiority of women.

Historically, in the structuring of society, men claimed authority and responsibility for the welfare of their families. In time however, authority took precedence over the welfare of the family. This change has contributed to spousal abuse and domestic violence.

Men do not need to define themselves as tough to express dominance. In general, men have difficulty expressing their feminine side and overplay their "macho-ness" by a show of force and violence. It is progressively more evident that men need to get in touch with their softer side to achieve a balance in masculine and feminine qualities. This shift to embrace the feminine side should be a cause for celebration as men are relieved from the "perceived" societal roles of protector and provider. They are free to grow and develop and realize their own full potential, with greater possibilities, freedoms and rewards. Being vulnerable is a human trait and not a weakness.

Increasingly, the patriarchal role is shown to be a non-sustaining model for a lasting and healthy relationship. Searching for a better model, we turn to creation myths. The origin and nature of being from non-being is often portrayed as the result of a sexual union. The two parents are commonly identified as male Sky and female Earth, neither playing the dominant role. In the Hindu account of creation, God was originally neither male nor female. Overcome by loneliness it divided itself into the male and the female, so each remained incomplete without the other. This theme of unity and duality is seen throughout India. The erotic statues are religious allegories of the perfect, indestructible union of the energies of the cosmos—Shiva, (the divine masculine aspect) and Shakti (the divine feminine creative power). There is a male-female interdependence, rather than a male mastery of the female.

Taking this cosmic perspective of unity, male and female complement and complete each other. The strength of one balancing and stabilizing the nurturing and compassion of the other. Men and women differ but like the yin / yang symbol, are as equal

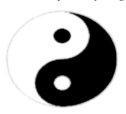

halves of the whole, each containing a "seed" or essence of the other. The smaller circles nested within each half of the symbol serve as a constant reminder of the interdependent nature of the black/white opposites. Both sides yielding and pushing into each other. The whole is greater than the two halves, continuously transforming, one into the other—different, and distinct. This is the new sustainable model for a healthy relationship and is best illustrated by this anonymous quote *"Don't walk behind me; I may not lead. Don't walk in front of me; I may not follow. Just walk beside me and be my friend."*

Each member of the partnership is autonomous in their own right but yet come together as one. Another parallel is that of the two overlapping rings that you see on wedding invitation cards.

This is the symbol of the Mandorla, or a Venn diagram. Mandorla is the Italian word for almond. It is an ancient symbol of two circles overlapping to form an almond shape in the middle—a place where the opposites of masculinity and femininity meet and honor one another.

The Mandorla is the container in which the new creation of the union of male and female begins to form the entity of "us." The area of the overlap is shared space but each ring has its own space. Each ring is complete in itself. The overlap may be very thin at first, like a sliver of a new moon. With maturing, forging and shaping, the overlap becomes greater. With the painful conflicts and contradictions of life, one can seek solace in the Mandorla, symbolizing the safe space of unity and interdependence.

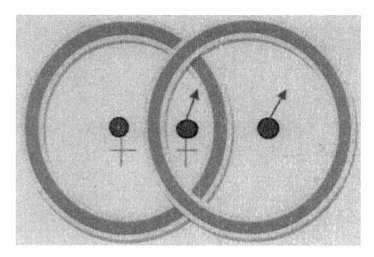

Mandorla of Relationship

Being in an intimate relationship means having another take a personal interest in you; someone that understands you just as much as you understand the other; success is shared and troubles halved. Love dies when there is violence, neglect or abandonment or if there is blame or over-dependency. Domination and over-possessiveness are also barriers to a healthy relationship. There needs to be realistic expectations of the other and an acceptance or compromise of differences. Having that intimate relationship means having a greater objective of living than the mere pleasing of self. Each is interested in the other's pleasure and welfare. Building a healthy intimacy requires ongoing communication of thought and feeling from a center of authenticity in an environment of stability and security.

Meditative Exercise

Find a quiet place, relax with the mindful breathing technique. Breathe in gently through the nose and breathe out with slow relaxed exhalations. Let the breath be as light as a feather. Enjoy the company of yourself.

With a single-mind, focus on your relationship; bring to mind the exhilaration you felt during the courting period. In this euphoric state, your happiness bubbled up and spilled over to everyone. You were flying high and all was right with the world during this honeymoon period. With time, the demands of daily living bring you down to face reality.

It is inevitable that disagreements and friction occur at such times. Be mindful of your needs as much as your partner's needs. All of us change and grow. Take time to ponder your differences and temper it with understanding and acceptance.

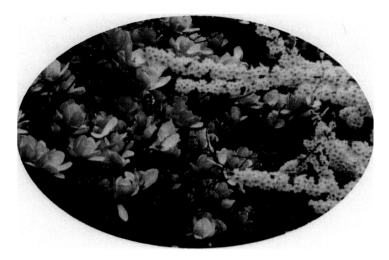

Backyard treasures

The beauty of one complementing the strength of the other. Understanding is the key to harmony and resolution of conflict. Be creative about the ways you can nourish the other and grow the Mandorla. Do this as a regular practice to strengthen the bonds of intimacy.

Chapter 12
AGES AND STAGES

"To every thing there is a season, and a time to every purpose under the heaven"
—Ecclesiastes 3:1 kjv

Childhood is a phase of life where growth and development occur at a pace that is not matched at any other time in life. The infant learns to recognize itself and its relationship to those who care for him/her. The young brain is absorbing input from the environment and learns to express itself. This is a stage in life where levels of sex hormones (ovarian or testicular) are low. Children are not physically, emotionally or socially adapted to adult sexual behaviors.

Adolescence is the period of transition. Hormonal levels fluctuate and increase. The adolescent becomes aware of body changes and development of breast and sexual organs. They often indulge in sex play and experimentation. Emotionally they transition from dependence to independence and distance themselves from parents or care givers.

The adult stage is a period of intense striving and activity. Hormone levels become cyclically stable. This is generally the period of sexuality, reproduction and caring for offspring. Fending for and supporting self and family becomes prime in importance.

Society has predestined that this adult stage of sexuality should last forever. Millions of dollars are spent in perpetuating and promoting "the sex" myth that all you need is to replace the hormones and you will have the same body and sexual functions of a young adult. The body does change, however, and hormones decrease after a certain age for a reason. Teilard de Chardin stated that all progress is made by passing through some stages of instability. This is the midlife "crisis" that gives us pause in the road map of our lives. There is a sense of an inner restlessness—a need to re-examine our past and reconsider and reclaim the future. Christiane Northrup speaks of the changes that occur with the menopause as *"the voice that insists on speaking up and leads to a sharper eye for inequity and injustice."* It holds true for the male equivalent of andropause.

But the good news is that this is a harbinger to a phase in life that expresses an emotional stability and greater maturity of thought.

The stage of the wise woman/man or crone/sage is a gift. This is the time for wisdom and individuation as there is no longer a pressing need for striving and long term goals.

Hormonal levels in the child are at a low level but yet childhood is a time of rapid growth and development. It therefore shreds the myth that it is the low levels of hormones that causes the slew of symptoms that hormonal supplementation allegedly would cure. This assumption of cause and effect is a huge medical mistake. It is an inaccuracy to credit the normal hormonal levels of a young adult to the later stages life. The societal drive to maintain a youthful appearance has led the pharmaceutical industry to push the concept of hormonal deficiency. If 100 percent of women have low levels of estrogen after a certain age, that is the norm and not a deficiency. Long term hormonal therapy during and after the menopause has now been shown to increase cardiac events as well as breast and uterine cancer. Because of the obstructive efforts of big pharma, the evidence for the harm of hormonal replacement therapy (HRT) was a long time coming.

Similarly, the pursuit for "power, performance and passion" in men has led to the T-drug (testosterone) craze. There is little data to support testosterone supplementation to reverse age related decline in males. A recent Time magazine feature article titled "Manopause" cites a whopping $2.4 billion in testosterone sales. It goes on to say that several studies had linked heart attacks and strokes with the use of testosterone. (Note the parallel to estrogen supplementation). Testosterone supplementation also increases testosterone dependent prostate diseases such as benign prostatic hypertrophy and prostate cancer.

With age, physical challenges to engage in sex may emerge. Spontaneity in sex may not be as predictable as we would like it to be. This does not mean that sex is "done" as we age, but rather that it takes a lesser role. We may find that we have to plan for it more. As death or illness claims a spouse, partners may not be physically or emotionally available. Children may be leaving the home but aged parents may be requiring challenging attention and care leaving one with less time and energy.

The natural decline of aging is not the effect of a single factor or hormone. To assume so is reductionism without substantiating facts. The endocrine glands, the hypothalamic-pituitary system, genes, culture, chronic or acute illness and a multitude of other factors play a role. We dream of the fountain of eternal youth, not appreciating the wellspring of maturity. Understanding and accepting the natural aging process, with physical and mental upkeep, we can find health and wellbeing.

In actuality, sex hormones start declining at the age of thirty. After the midlife, there is a reversal of the pubescent changes, as reproduction is no longer nature's intention. The body changes and adapts to the changing roles we play. Breast and reproductive organs shrink. Hormonal fluctuations and decline lead to physical symptoms of hot flashes and insomnia in women and restlessness in men. This "midlife crisis" is a period where there needs to be a meno/andro "pause" and time taken to reevaluate and reassess one's values and goals. This period that can "feel like death" is a rite of passage directed inward.

The passing of what is valued in youth allows for the birth of new possibilities in the years ahead. The higher cortical functions play a more major role as we mature and provide a wider and more experiential view of life. Greater satisfaction, joy and fulfillment are found in companionship, music, art, creativity, and /or spirituality. Leadership and teaching roles may become more predominant. Successful aging involves a willingness to leave behind that which is "done with;" to allow the blossoming of creative potential and to embrace the new responsibilities of guide and mentor.

Medical Applications

We need to use medications responsibly. The risks and benefits have to be weighed individually. Women go through a difficult time during the menopause due the chaotic fluctuations of hormonal levels. Hormonal therapy may be used during this trying period to even out the fluctuations and phased out in one to two years for a gentle let down. It is essential to use science and technology responsibly and with integrity to help rather than manipulate the public for corporate financial gain.

Meditative Exercise

Dress appropriately for the weather. Find a peaceful walking path that you enjoy.

As you place one foot in front of the other feel the solidity of the earth beneath you... Feel the movement of air with its life giving oxygen ruffling your hair and caressing your face. Breathe in the peace of your surroundings and breathe out gently letting the out-breath be a little longer than the in-breath.

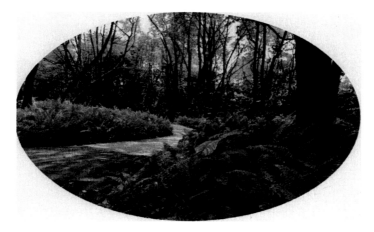

Hort Park Singapore

Soak in the beauty of trees and plants on your walk—the greenery that sucks up the toxic carbon dioxide that we breathe out. Picture a caterpillar on a leaf. Ponder on the stages of its life, withdrawing into a cocoon and then emerging into a butterfly.

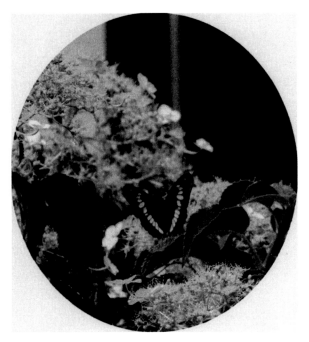

Each phase complete in itself, having its time and place in the universe. Reflect on your life's journey. Think back to your childhood, the teenage years and adult life. Each stage merges into the other to form a complete whole. Re-evaluate priorities and aspirations for the future.

CHAKRA 3

SOLAR PLEXUS CHAKRA
TEN PETALS OF THE EMOTIONS (LIGHT & DARK)

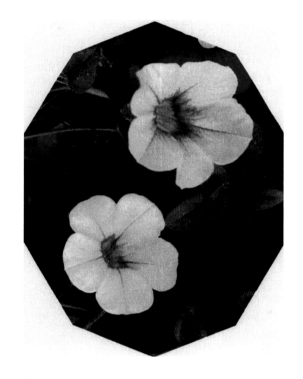

Love
Joy
Awe
Trust
Acceptance

Hate
Grief
Greed
Fear
Anger

Chapter 13
TEN PETALS OF THE EMOTIONS

"Emotions in life are like wild horses that have to be reined in by the charioteer."

—Plato

"I don't want to be at the mercy of my emotions. I want to use them, to enjoy them, and to dominate them."
—Oscar Wilde, *The Picture of Dorian Gray*

The location of the third chakra is at the level of the solar or coeliac plexus above the navel and below the chest. It is the chakra of the emotions. The color of the third Chakra is yellow, a primary color in the artist's palette. Yellow is the color of ripe lemons, tart and biting; and daffodils, the color of sunshine and joy. Bright yellow is an attention getting color, a call for action.

Emotions serve a purpose in humans (and lower species) in aiding in their survival and avoiding danger. Psychologist Silvan Tomkins' research into affect finds that emotion is necessary to motivate behavior.

We can think of "emotion" as a merge of the two words: emote (which is to feel) and motion. There is a subjective feeling with a physiological physical reaction, followed by a behavioral response to the emotion. Emotions are an alert system that prepares one to make a decision. Emotions are crucial in how we think and behave. They are part of the organizing forces in our lives. This chakra is the basis of the fight/flight/freeze/flop or figure it out reactions.

Emotions are present in all animals and humans to varying degrees. An understanding of the ways that we are similar as well as different from animals gives us appreciation of what it means to be human. Emotions are ingrained as a prefabricated template or cookie cutter that is genetically set for each species. All humans are capable of feeling any and all of the spectrum of human emotions. It is not a failing to have any of these feelings.

Infants within the first week of life are able to read the expressions on their mother's faces. Anthropologists have determined that facial expressions of emotion are universal across human cultures and thus biological in origin and not culturally determined. It allows one to feel out the inner states and motives of those around us and prepares us physically to respond. Emotions are the social sense organ. It is a means to communicate with others and for others to understand us to build deeper meaningful relationships. Being able to correctly define another's emotions is a valuable skill that can be developed. People bond together with an emotional resonance as they share their feelings. Unfortunately, internal emotions do not always correlate with outward expression. And negative feelings can be spread to large groups, inciting hatred, anger and violence.

All emotions do not have a value, they are neither good nor bad. They just are. What gives the emotion value is the *effect* on oneself and on others. The value judgment is secondary to culture, society and upbringing. One never has to justify or be ashamed of a feeling but one may regret or be ashamed of the actions that follow.

> *"Between the emotion and the response lies the shadow"*
> —T.S. Elliot, "The Hollow Men"

The value of the emotion can also be dependent on the situation. We are likely to feel grief if we broke something of value ourselves but if someone else broke it we are more apt to anger.

The Hebrew Bible indicates that humanity was formed with two impulses: a good impulse (the yetzer tov) and an evil impulse (the yetzer ra). The Chinese yin/yang symbol similarly emphasizes this duality of the nature of man. A Cherokee legend tells the story of the battle between two wolves—the battle of good and evil within. The one that wins is the one that is fed. Bertrand Russell in his autobiography envisioned a utopia where individuals are free; where hate, greed and envy die because there is nothing there to nourish them.

Motivators or triggers for an emotion can be an external event or an internal stimulus that is derived from past memory, or a thought related to a current or future event. Life stressors, unmet expectations and needs, disappointments or mood of the people around you play a part in the emotion aroused. Relatively insignificant events can trigger or escalate the original emotional response.

Essentially all emotions are processed in the mid brain (the "feeling brain") and if we allow it, the higher cortical centers modify the reaction. Perception, thinking, memory and action are involved in the expression of emotions. There is a close interaction between brain and body systems to sense and feel, and then think and act.

Exactly how firing of neurons in the brain translates an experience into an emotion is largely unknown. What we do know is that the stimulus is processed in the amygdala (part of the limbic system or primitive brain) where the emotion is "perceived" or "generated." All animals have a limbic system: for aggression, to find food; for love, to have and care for their offspring; and for fear, to avoid threatening situations. The initial emotion tends to be short lasting, an instantaneous reaction to a stimulus.

From the amygdala the impulse is sent to the hypothalamus which relays information to the sympathetic or parasympathetic systems, the endocrine glands and/or to the motor systems for action. Simultaneously, impulses are sent to the higher cortical centers, which being farther away, take a little longer to process. The higher cortical centers bring awareness to the episode and allow the thinking brain to execute decision making. This is where humans differ from animals. We have a larger and more developed frontal cortex to modify our limbic reactions.

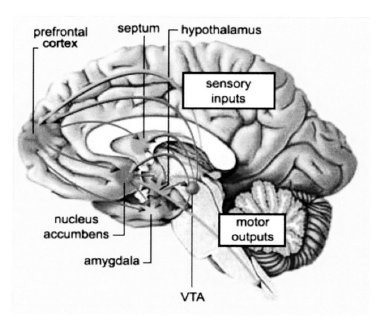

Limbic System
Wikimedia: The Brain from Top to Bottom under copyleft

The amygdala (*yellow*) is a major constituent of the emotion-producing limbic system (*light blue*). And the hypothalamus (*orange*), in response to signals from the prefrontal cortex, amygdala and hippocampus, directs the release of hormones that support motor responses to perceived threats.

Although the initial emotion is short lasting, the threshold for activating that emotion is lowered. If another trigger arises, the emotion is activated faster and more intensely. Not uncommonly, the emotion stays "stuck" in the mind because of reinforcements from past memory and a succession of recurring thoughts. In other words, thoughts and memories perpetuate, magnify and prolong the emotion.

In the book the *Life of Pi*, emotions are represented as the tiger, Richard Parker. Like Pi, one needs to need to tame/gain control of/develop a relationship with this "emotion" center of the brain. So often the mind locks us into the negative feeling, feeding into it and fanning the flames. We can work on self-regulatory strategies by changing our thoughts related to the incident, and reduce the intensity and duration of negative emotions. Emotional intelligence is being consciously aware of our emotional state without becoming overwhelmed or consumed by it. Once we become aware of our emotion, there is a split second to allow conscious choice to alter or change the reflex reaction. Hence the adage—" count to ten before speaking or acting." Every feeling can be arrested if we place awareness, or shine a light on it, before we act on it irrationally.

To be fully human, we need to embrace our complete range of emotions. Feelings surge like the tide—unstoppable. But we can choose to ride the tide or step aside.

The spectrum of emotions seen in humans, like colors on a palette, can have shades and combinations. To put it in another way, the range of human emotions can be compared to a kaleidoscope that changes its appearance with a tiny shift or tilt.

Plutchik's cone (or wheel) of emotions is an excellent artistic rendering of the scope of human emotions. The cone divides emotions into eight main feelings that are graded in severity. Combinations give rise to sub emotions.

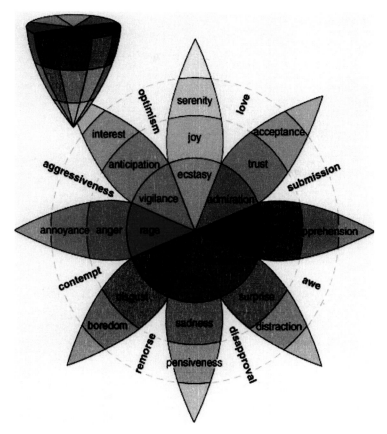

Plutchik's Wheel/Cone of Emotions
Author: Ivan Akira
Source: Wikimedia commons
License: Creative Commons Attribution 3.0 Unported

All emotions need to be acknowledged as they are flags for action. What we value as good emotions have been shown to have a positive influence on all cells of the body, mind and spirit. Positive emotions enhance immune functions through the T cells (which are white blood cells that manage immune defenses) and killer cells (white blood cells that destroy infected or cancer cells).

All that we feel becomes deeply ingrained in our tissues and our psyche. Persistent and sustained negative emotions have a detrimental effect that harms tissues. It has been shown that hostility and anxiety lead to high blood pressure and heart attacks. Working on cultivating positive emotions by feeding them enhances health.

A simple exercise to prove this point is to close one's eyes and focus on an event that brought out anger in you. Feel the tightening of muscles around the throat, constriction around the heart and tension in the body. Let go of this emotion and come back to the moment. Next imagine a situation that was joyful—like surfing the waves or feeling the ocean breeze in your hair. Feel the warmth and relaxation and a sense of well-being that follows.

Because emotions and physical health are interrelated, understanding the emotions and making better choices in response to them makes for a more healthy and wholesome life. For my purpose, I have modified Plutchik's wheel to ten basic emotions to reflect the ten petals of the third chakra; trust and fear, joy and grief, love and hate, acceptance and anger, awe and greed.

According to research by Glasgow University all human behavior can be reduced to four basic core emotions—mad, sad, glad and scared. As all emotions involve the limbic system, an understanding of every feeling will evolve as I elaborate on these four core sentiments.

Chapter 14
FEAR

Our deepest fear is that we are powerful beyond meas-
ure. It is our light, not our darkness that most frightens
us…As we're liberated from our own fear, Our presence
automatically liberates others.
—Marianne Williamson in "A Return to Love"

"Even death is not to be feared by one who has lived
wisely"

—Buddha

Fear is a basic, innate emotion in response to a stimulus or threat
of danger. Fear and anger are two sides of the same coin. Fear
underpins anger and is generated from the same flight/fight response system in the body. Fear leads to retreat from the situation
while anger leads one to attack. Fear is associated with the expec-
tation that something destructive will happen to us. Fear is a survival strategy that allows one to avoid danger. Excessive fear,
however, can lead one to freeze or to panic.

On the other hand, if there is no personal threat involved, the fear response can be a stimulating and pleasurable event. This is the draw of horror and adventure films that keep us on the edge of our seats gnawing at our finger nails. Facing and transcending a fearful situation can be exhilarating and accounts for athletes engaging in extreme sports such as sky diving. Fear-based challenges enable us to push the envelope and explore new horizons.

An animal's ability to experience fear triggers the flight/freeze response and is essential for its survival. The angry mother bird attacks the predator to protect the young ones in her care. Fear allows the animal to run away from danger.

Connections from the amygdala to hypothalamic and brainstem sites explain many of the observed signs of conditioned fear responses. The amygdala, interacts with the hypothalamus triggering a cascade of neurochemicals and hormones leading to increased sweating, trembling and a rapid heartbeat, (see diag. pg. 125, substituting instant fight/anger with instant flight/fear reaction). Breathing speeds up; pupils dilate to see better; metabolism of fat and glucose in the liver increase to provide the energy that is needed to escape from danger. The decision-making centers in the neocortex need time to assess and appropriately regulate the nature and duration of the response. Because the amygdala is aroused before the neocortex can accurately assess the situation, one experiences the physical effects of fear even in the case of a false alarm or a memory of a traumatic experience. The hippocampus, by retrieving these traumatic memories, links the thinking brain (neocortical areas) to the feeling brain (limbic system). and sets in motion the fear response.

The brain has the ability to change its response and reactions. Nerve cells pass signals to each other and to their target organs by releasing messenger molecules, called transmitters. There are at least thirty known transmitters in the brain and billions of neurons and trillions of synapses which account for the myriads of responses possible and why we can learn to change our response. Fear feeds on itself and depends on the attention we give it. By renaming the fear we can transform it to have empowerment for positive action. Fear can be fuel for creativity and passion.

"Do the thing you fear most and the death of fear is certain"
—Mark Twain.

Buddhism lists Five Great Fears: fear of death, fear of illness (especially cancer), fear of losing your mind, fear of loss of livelihood, and fear of public speaking writes Lewis Richmond in *Aging as a Spiritual Practice*.

Fear of death is often what underlies most fears. Death is an ever present reality and an inevitable conclusion of life. There is no escape from it. Often it is the sudden death of someone close that brings this home. Premature death and some illnesses, on the other hand, can be minimized by following holistic principles of healthy living and reducing unhealthy habits. Gene D Cohen in his book *The Mature Mind* emphasizes that events promoting a balanced emotional response, lead to positive changes in the body, as there is an interconnection between brain and body through nerves, hormones and the immune system. Only by facing the reality of death and illness and acknowledging one's mortality can one live life to the fullest.

Dame Cicely Saunders, founder of the hospice movement died of cancer, as she wished, at age eighty-seven at a hospice she founded. Her wish was to die of cancer as it would give her time to express her regrets, thank those she needed to and say her final goodbyes. She faced the reality of her death with practical action.

Fear can be conscious or unconscious and can be imposed by society and family. Walls of fear can stem from ignorance toward others not like us. It may be related to sexual orientation, race or religion. Politicians and the media often build up a culture of fear, manipulating words by selection or omission of facts and distortion of statistics. The stigmatization of minorities—such as African Americans, Native Americans, Jews in the forties, women, and gays—has led to unprecedented carnage and grief. Fear springs from our ignorance and weaknesses.

The Buddhist Canon lists five mental strengths to deal with fear: discernment, persistence, conviction, concentration, and mindfulness.

Concentration and mindfulness provides the mind with a still center and teaches us to focus our attention, not on the object of our fear, but on fear as a mental event. With mindfulness we stop drowning in or identifying with the fear. We gain strength, courage and confidence by every experience in which we really stop to look fear in the face. By persistently building on our strengths and honestly exploring the issues we face, we can sweep away the cobwebs of unrealistic fears. Being aware of these important learning moments we can choose a more positive strategy rather than denial, worry or panic.

If we can overcome fear, we put ourselves in a position of strength. Seeing shadows in the darkness brings terror and fear. But as we walk toward it and see the shadow for what it is, the fear melts away. Creepy sounds in the night makes hair stand on end; but by investigating the source of the sound we may recognize it for the scratching of a tree branch on the window pane and know that our fear was unfounded. The delusions surrounding our fears can cause us to misconstrue the dangers we face, seeing danger where there is none. Only when we develop mental strengths can we see through the delusions that give fear its power. We can shift gears to a position where we are no longer threatened by that fear ever again. By training the mind we can work with the emotion as it arises. We can examine it and break it into its component parts. By doing so we can understand it better and not let it overcome us. We can only experience one emotion at any one moment. Fear being the stronger emotion blocks out joy. The ability to choose a positive perspective leads to greater happiness and satisfaction in life. In other words—change your thoughts and in so doing, change your life.

Medical Applications

Persistently allowing the limbic system to take over the cortical regulatory system can lead to pathological conditions such as anxiety, panic attacks, phobia, paranoia, or post-traumatic stress disorder. Whatever the fear, whether it is fear of loneliness, conflict, betrayal, or decision making, take time to mull over it. Face the issue and make choices based on facts as far as possible. Mistakes are generally correctable and it is usually possible to chart a new course.

Emotional memories are reactivated when a fearful event is recalled. This vulnerable state is the window of opportunity to change the memory of that experience. Changing thoughts associated with the event during this time changes the stored memory. A sense of purpose and meaning can thus be re-established. Reappraising how we interpret a stressful occurrence can suppress the fear response—a technique described as reframing.

Another coping strategy is to strengthen cortical input by naming the emotion. By bringing the fear into awareness, the cortical centers are activated and the amygdala response is suppressed. Experience, learning and repetition bolster the connections between amygdala and pre-frontal control centers. This is the basis of cognitive psychotherapy especially helpful for post-traumatic stress disorder (PTSD) transforming it to post-traumatic growth.

Meditative Exercise

Prepare yourself for meditation by settling in a position of comfort, whether it is laying down or sitting cross legged on the floor or in a chair. Start with slow relaxed breathing as before. Focus on a fear that you are facing. Observe the myriad thoughts that surface in relation to this fear. Observe the thoughts with detachment, not judging or reacting.

Indian ocean/Sri Lanka

Label your fear treating it as nothing more than objects of attention, like dolphins in the deep, blue sea. Being a detached witness of your thoughts allows you to distance yourself from the emotion and thereby, through self-awareness, modulate your reactions. Experience the shift that occurs as you separate yourself from the destructive whirlpool of the mind.

Breathe gently into this new awareness with gratitude.

Chapter 15
ANGER

He that is slow to anger is better than the mighty; and he that ruleth his spirit than he that taketh a city.
—Proverbs 16:32 kjv

"Holding onto anger is like grasping a hot coal with the intent of throwing it at someone else. You are the one who gets burned."

—The Buddha

Reportedly there are twenty-seven different levels of anger. It ranges from a mild feeling of impatience, irritability or grouchiness to an intense rage that builds up and explodes often with violence.

Emotion is innate but the emotional reaction is learned behavior. When buttons get pushed, we react automatically. Our immediate behavior usually reflects the emotional survival program existing considerably below our conscious mind. Our behavior is instantaneous without forethought, deliberation or discretion. Just as any animal by nature, when faced with a sudden sound or movement, instinctively tenses all its muscles to prepare for fight, flight, or freeze, so do we humans instantly react to a perceived threat. Anger occurs at the preconscious level, instantaneously and unbidden. The primitive brain has preempted our rational self. Knowing this we can accept and acknowledge the feeling of anger when it arises without blame or guilt.

We can find a non-harmful way to acknowledge and express the feeling. We can deal with the anger by talking or writing about it, or find a safe place to vent and feel understood. We can harness the anger and transform the feeling to a meaningful and constructive action. Or we can give way to aggressive or violent behavior. We can accept this invitation to anger and make the choice to build or destroy. According to Ronald Potter Efron, we can be *"consciously selective so you don't waste your energy on trivial matters. Rate the importance—from trivial to life threatening and seek a balanced perspective."*

Confronted by someone or something perceived as potentially harmful we're desperate to squash that threat as quickly as we can. The compelling force to vigorously defend oneself is a primitive operating system. It does not offer time to consider the *consequences* of our impetuous reactions. No time is spent to reflect on the most effective response to the offending person or event. This is where "all hell can break loose." But **as** humans it is our choice to fight, flee, freeze, or to figure it out for mutual gain.

It takes half a second for the amygdala to be activated by an emotional trigger. Incoming information is processed at the unconscious level and leads to bodily responses through the sympathetic (arousal) systems. Additionally, adrenaline and cortisol are released through the endocrine system through the hypothalamus and adrenals. These stress hormones, speed up our heart rate and breathing and give us a burst of energy. Blood pressure also rises as our blood vessels constrict. These bodily responses mobilize us for emergencies and are an integral part of the emotional process to prepare for the "fight or flight" response.

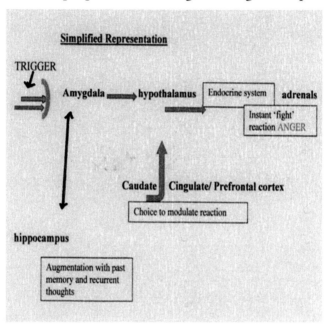

The amygdala also has connections to the hippocampus that is the center for memory. The Hippocampus, part of limbic system, connects emotions and senses to form new memories, sorts and catalogs memories and sends them to the cerebral cortex for long term memory storage. It also retrieves memory when needed and feeds it back to the amygdala.

The mind creates a sense of continuity, linking past experiences with the present perceptions and anticipation of future events. Memories of past scenes and repeated experiences shape responses. Inflexible patterns of thinking repeat the cycle and the same pattern of response emerges. So past experiences, similar to or related to the provocation (that may be perceived rather than real) can cause us to react in deeply ingrained ways to reinforce the anger. Ruminating on the hurt contributes to the spiraling anger and adds to the suffering. With habitual patterns of anger, the anger is triggered more rapidly, lasts longer with each episode, and becomes more intense.

A person who has grown up in a family where violence was the norm of family life might have a harder time controlling anger and is more likely to act out violently. Because of their upbringing, this person who acts aggressively or violently may believe that violence is the only way to deal with anger and may not have the skills to act in any other way. These behavior patterns may lead to changes in DNA which passes to the offspring, perpetuating the cycle of violence.

The good news is that in humans, with the development of the neocortex and higher brain structures it is possible to break through this vicious cycle by conscious awareness. The amygdala sends and receives information to the caudate nucleus, cingulate gyrus and the medial prefrontal cortex. This brings the feeling into awareness and allows for a more rational and thoughtful response. There is a two to three second interval before the prefrontal cortex receives the information from the amygdala for a more considerate, sensible decision. Knowing this, we can learn to take a few deep breaths or count to ten before reacting. Anger is in the word danger. It is a red flag to a bull. So when you see red, wait at the amber light before you "go" at green. It takes patience and mental retraining to wait with the tension of the anger and not seek an immediate resolution.

Harville Hendrix who developed *"imago couples* therapy counsels his clients to mirror and validate statements made so that both parties are on the same page and what is said is what is understood. This helps to clarify perceptions before reaction and lengthens the gap between impulse and action. By mirroring, we buy time to make decisions and actions that are informed by our emotions and not controlled by them. It gives time for the cortical processes to be activated. With greater self-awareness we can modulate our responses with care. With cognitive control, comes authentic power.

We generally get angry and become overly caught up with thought processes and emotions in response to perceived threat. The threat may be a current event or an anticipatory thought and it may be colored/reinforced by history. An insult, violations of core values or injustice (toward ourselves or others dear to us) could be real or imagined. Albert Ellis rightly states that no person or thing could—in and of themselves—cause us to react a particular way because it's always our *interpretation* of the outside stimulus that finally governs our reaction to it.

It's critical to identify just what pushes our buttons. Anything powerful enough to have pushed our buttons previously is quite likely to push them again. When we lack awareness, we get pulled into the emotion which consumes us. The trigger isn't necessarily something that would provoke someone else. Identifying and recognizing our triggers or 'hot buttons' is the key to emotional control. We can become more aware of them by naming them.

Often this hot button relates to getting criticized, rejected or undervalued, disapproved or humiliated, or unfairly treated, or taken advantage of, or our integrity is questioned.

Don Miguel Ruiz in "The Four Agreements" gives invaluable advice in his second agreement. He offers that what others say and do is a projection of their own reality and not to take things personally. Their needs (or values) are just as legitimate and meaningful to them as one's own. When one is open to the opinions and actions of others, one is less likely to react. Seeing the situation as the other's failings rather than a personal affront helps to step back and take stock and see things from a fresh perspective.

Think about being tough on the issue, and soft on the person, to solve problems without blame for self or other. It is important to direct the anger towards the problem rather than the person, focusing on answers and constructive ways to solve differences. We can learn to separate the person we are relating to, and the issue or behavior being addressed.

It also helps, in retrospect, to picture how we could have handled the situation differently. How, for instance, the next time we can refrain from "taking the bait" or feel obligated to defend ourselves against criticism. This demands insight, emotional poise, and interpersonal skills.

Medical Applications

Anger and hostility release the stress hormones which causes harm if activated repeatedly. Studies suggest that high blood pressure may be associated with both extremes of emotional behavior, either always suppressing anger or always expressing it overtly. High cortisol and high adrenaline levels is cardio toxic. Persistent elevation of the three major stress hormones cortisol, adrenaline and epinephrine can damage blood vessels and arteries, increasing blood pressure and raising the risk of heart attacks or strokes. It is also associated with sleep and memory problems, exhaustion and lack of concentration.

With anger and resentment, our stomach tenses and digestion is impaired and contributes to ulcers and irritable bowel syndrome. Crippling arthritis, fibromyalgia and chronic fatigue syndrome may be associated with chronic anger.

Unresolved anger results in anxiety and mood disturbances. We are more likely to be disagreeable and argumentative and be wary of everyone, not just the offending person. To protect ourselves from further hurt we push others away and become emotionally isolated, empty and depressed. It robs us of joy and peace as we lose our enthusiasm for hobbies and passions and withdraw from social activities. This ultimately reflects back on work and career.

The use of drugs and alcohol is often associated with a tendency to anger and violent behavior as self-awareness and cognitive control are lost.

Meditative Exercise

Find a comfortable, quiet spot whether it is in the home or out in nature under a shady tree. Start by closing the eyes and center with slow, relaxed breathing.

Imagine a river that is flowing by. A storm starts up and the river starts to rage and swirl. The storm gets stronger and the raging river becomes a torrent of energy, wreaking havoc in its path, hurling rocks and eroding the river bed. You are the swirling river. You are the energy of anger. Anger is in you and is you. The hurling rocks are your angry, recurrent thoughts hurting you. Let go and disengage from these destructive thoughts. They are merely creations of your mind.

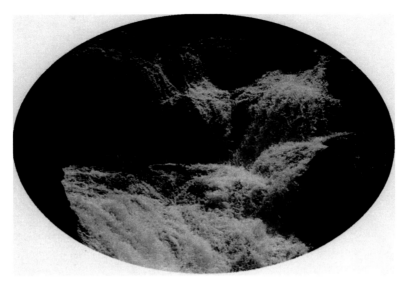

Dunn's River Falls, Jamaica

Let the storm pass and let the river resume its calm. The water is clear and you see the river bed with its stunning, myriad life forms. You see the under-water vegetation. You see colorful fish swimming peacefully, darting between the rocks and plant life. This is your mind. Your mind is calm. You see with clarity and purpose. You can step out of the raging water to the calmness and clarity of mind. This is your choice.

Come back to your breath and back to the quiet spot armed with tools to cope with anger.

Chapter 16
GRIEF AND LOSS

"Do not stand at my grave and weep. I am not there, I do not sleep I am a thousand winds that blow, I am the diamond glints on snow. I am the sunlight on ripened grain, I am the gentle autumn's rain."

—Mary Frye

Loss is the experience of having something or someone to which you have formed a bond or attachment taken away from you. Grief is the feeling associated with the loss. Grief is an emotion that is seen even in animals. Donna Fernandes describes seeing a gorilla say good-bye to his longtime mate Babs who had died of cancer. She said that the gorilla was howling and banging his chest and trying to feed Babs to get her to wake up. Jane Goodall observed Flint, a young chimpanzee, withdraw from his group, stop eating, and die of a broken heart after the death of his mother, Flo.

Mourning is the process of expression for the loss. The way one mourns or expresses grief is dependent on culture, family history, social and religious influences, temperament, and strength of the attachment or love. Mourning allows one to work through the loss and make meaning of it. Rituals of mourning may serve to strengthen the social bonds among the survivors who band together to pay their last respects. In India, families gather at the funeral pyre along the sacred Ganges River and chant for the release of their loved one's soul at the time of the cremation. In Western cultures, a wake or viewing, is conducted for friends and family.

Most religions offer a concept of life after death to assuage anxiety associated with loss. Hinduism and Buddhism promote reincarnation. Islam and Christianity extol Paradise as an after-life place of abundance and beauty, following the last judgment for the life lived on earth. The Admiralty Islanders believe that the dead coexist with the living in a different mode of being and so did the ancient Greeks and Romans.

The notion of heaven and the life to come possibly dis-counts present life. Also, the concept of judgment day may fill one with worry, self-doubt and guilt over the life lived. Eckhart Tolle astutely states that believing in a future heaven can create a present hell.

China and Japan ritualize existence after death and send ob-jects of comfort with the dear departed. When a Hmong person dies his or her soul must travel back in time and space to the bur-ial place of its placenta ("birth jacket") and only after it is properly dressed in this finest of clothing can it continue on its journey to be reunited with its ancestors.

Stoic philosophy encourages acceptance of things that cannot be changed. If someone should die, those close to them should keep their serenity because the loved one, made of flesh and blood, was destined to death. Death is not feared as people do not "lose" their life, but instead "return" to the source.

Questions about the nature of death have plagued us since the beginning of civilization. Human cultures have sensed a reality of life beyond time and space through their myths and religious beliefs. Socrates states *"Either death is a state of nothingness and utter unconsciousness, or, as men say, there is a change and migration of the soul from this world to another."* Modern science claims that the brain creates consciousness. And therefore awareness ceases to exist with death of the brain.

The closest we have come to knowing what is out there after life is in the experiences of those who have had near death experiences (NDE). People with NDE are generally more empathic and intuitive after their experience. They become motivated to live life more fully, seeing life as a gift and celebrating it rather than living with the fear of death. We lose the meaning of life when we are too preoccupied with death and whatever lies beyond.

Whatever the beliefs regarding death and the afterlife, the pain of loss is easier to bear by internalizing the continuity of life and the inevitability of change and death. Native Americans say that every human being is born with a finite number of days to their circle of life. But each life, whether short or long is complete.

A flower dies to bring forth the seed which in turn gives rise to a new plant. Dead leaves of a tree are shed and new ones sprout. Surface cells of the body go through death and renewal every second. In grieving, we are acknowledging the death of what no longer exists.

As a culture, we generally discourage the direct expression of grief and all things associated with it. We often judge the one actively grieving and expressing pain by saying they are "not coping well." We attempt to cheer him or her and rationalize saying "You have to be brave for the children" or "You are doing so well," when they are not outwardly showing grief. But the intense, overwhelming emotion of grief is a natural, biological phenomenon likened to falling off a cliff edge into the churning currents of a whirlpool. You are battered against the rocks of heartache, sleeplessness and lethargy. All orientation, direction and support is lost.

Viewing grief as a natural part of our human experience allows one to express the pain of loss and to allow its natural course to play out. Psychiatrist Elisabeth Kubler-Ross describes five stages of emotional response in the course of grieving—denial, anger, bargaining, depression and acceptance—as normal responses to loss. These stages may be extrapolated to any kind of loss or disappointments, including a job loss or loss of a pet. All of these stages may not necessarily be expressed and may occur in random order.

From an evolutionary standpoint, grief serves to ensure that the partner or infant or thing is protected and taken care of. Grief is the price of love and is inevitable with meaningful attachments. The deeper the love the greater the grief. With the severing of that love that was a source of joy and comfort, we experience the painful separation and express sorrow for ourselves. With the shattering of close ties, we experience a double loss as a part of us also dies. We fear the future without our loved one; feelings of emptiness, despair, insecurity and loneliness overwhelm us.

The complex feelings associated with loss are connected with the limbic system as the natural adaptive response of the body. The initial neurobiological response to the loss leads to increases in catecholamine leading to anger. Secondarily, loss is associated with a lowered secretion of pleasure chemicals of dopamine and oxytocin; this leads to withdrawal, isolation and depression. Recurring thoughts from the prefrontal cortex potentiate the emotions of anger, guilt, and regret. Staying stuck with these repetitive thoughts can easily spiral one into the quicksand of clinical depression.

Grief is as individual as thumbprints. There is generally a period of being in limbo between the old routines before finding the new life and new attachments. Acceptance is the key to moving through and looking forward to reclaiming life anew. Ride the roller coaster of ups and downs. Embrace the down times. Allow moments of laughter and joy without guilt. By our trust and willingness to allow the ending, we open ourselves to a new beginning.

> *"Not to make loss beautiful, but to make loss the place where beauty starts. Where the heart understands for the first time the nature of its journey."*
> —Gregory Orr.

Medical Applications
Loss forces a change in one's life. Take the time and space to feel what is right for you and what you need without judgement. Express grief in ways that is comfortable for you whether it is through support groups, journaling, art forms, or a nature walk.

A family member, friend or a therapist can create a safe haven that can promote healing and growth through loss.

Understanding the body responses of grief as a natural, biological phenomenon, we can have compassion for and be tender to one going through the prolonged, intense physical and emotional pain of loss.

The hospice movement was started as a response to the terminally ill, recognizing that patients should have a choice and the ability to participate in the decisions that affect their destiny. The goal is to treat each dying person with dignity and compassion, and to improve the quality of life towards the end. We can also treat every person with dignity and compassion without waiting till the end of life to show it.

Living will documents, although not foolproof, offer a way to have one's preferences known regarding end of life issues. It reduces futile procedures which is the default in the medical system. Having a well-informed relative or friend as a legal advocate ensures that your wishes are more likely to be carried out should you become incapacitated through illness or injury. Face end of life issues head-on, understand the different aspects of life-prolonging measures, and be clear about communicating your wishes. Should you choose not to communicate your desires, the burden and guilt rests upon the family, often leading to family squabbles.

Meditative Exercise

The end of a life is inevitably associated with sadness. It brings us face to face with our own mortality.

Settle into your comfortable relaxed pose. Let your breath be calm and even. Let the in-breath be as long as the out-breath. Let there be a pause between the in-breath and out-breath. As you pause at this in-between space, appreciate the stillness.

Imagine yourself at the ocean's edge. Feel the gentle waves lapping at your bare feet. Feel the salty spray from the breakers on your cheeks. See the fluffy clouds gently shifting and changing in the blue of the sky. The ocean, the spray, the clouds, snow, and hailstones—all one as different forms of the same. Ponder deeply on the nature of things. Reflect on what the cycle of life and death means to you. Celebrate the mystery of life. Worrying about the end of life robs us of the fragrance of today. Learn from those who have been at the edge.

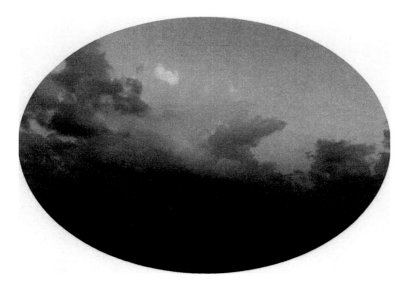

The Caribbean Ocean

Live each day as a precious gift.

Chapter 17
LOVE

Being deeply loved by someone gives you strength, Loving someone deeply gives you courage.

—Lao Tzu

Love is a basic universal human emotion, but understanding how and why it happens is not necessarily easy. It is an emotion that makes us happy or glad. Romantic and maternal love are evolutionary biological functions linked to the perpetuation of the species. It is associated with the release of hormones such as dopamine, norepinephrine, serotonin and oxytocin; and linked with the reward system of the brain. In other words these activities are designed to bring euphoria, to ensure that mating and mothering occurs. The activation of the hormones also lead to physical symptoms such as increased heart rate, loss of appetite and sleep—acutely experienced during the courting period and satirized in plays. People in love experience a kind of high that often lead to depression when feelings are not reciprocated.

The euphoria of love and its rewarding effects involve processes and pathways of the brain's limbic motivation and reward circuits. It seems that a part of the brain known as the Ventral Tegmental area (VTA), located in the midbrain at the top of the brainstem, is a center for cells that make dopamine (see diagram, pg. 85, & illus. pg. 111). The VTA connects to many areas of the brain including the caudate nucleus and hippocampus that results in feelings of elation and love. Brain scans confirm that parts of the caudate nucleus (a large, C-shaped region that sits deep near the center of the brain and situated over the sides of the limbic system) become active as a lover gazes at the photograph of a loved one. The frontal cortex by its connections to the caudate nucleus directs and executes behavior that achieves the goal of securing this love. In addition, regions of the brain associated with judgment and objectivity are deactivated. Reason goes out of the window when one is in love.

So what is love? The diversity of uses and meanings combined with the complexity of the feelings involved makes "love" difficult to consistently define. The concept is also limited by language, as the word love encompasses such a wide spectrum of emotions ranging from liking to ecstasy. Also the object of affection can be an inanimate thing, food, person or "God." C.S. Lewis, in his book *The Four Loves*, expands on this theme. Ancient Greeks identified four forms of love: kinship (storge), friendship (philia), sexual and/or romantic desire (eros), and divine love (agape). Agape love being a state of being and not an emotion will not be elaborated here but in a subsequent chapter.

Storge—Parental love involves care and responsibility necessary for the preservation of the child's life and growth. This love is unconditional and persists throughout the life of the child. Strong parent/child bonds serve to keep the infant close to the parent, and form a secure base for the child to venture out and explore the world. Parents impart guidance, discipline and guards them against threats increasing the chances of survival. Storge allows for a healthy environment for the child to develop socially, intellectually and emotionally, an impact that continues throughout life. Substitute parents generally tend to care less for children than natural parents and these children are more likely to be exploited or at risk.

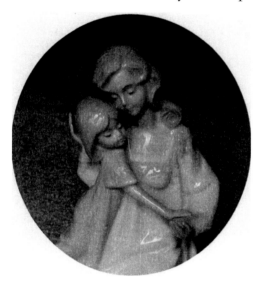

Brain scans show that children who were nurtured early in life showed a larger hippocampus. The hippocampus is crucial for learning, memory and response to stress: implying that a nurtured child is better suited to face life.

The emotional bond amongst family members is a bond that should be treasured and cultivated. "Blood runs thicker than water," it is said. In general, having a family member to count on in times of trouble cannot be underrated. Siblings often go the extra mile for each other when the need arises.

Philia expresses emotions between friends, companions or colleagues and includes the love for one's pets. This friendship is the strong bond existing between people who share common interests or activities. Passionate love is often born out of this familiarity.

Friends generally share attitudes, values and interests. There is mutual trust with the ability to be oneself, to express one's feelings, and make mistakes without fear of judgment. This allows for genuine enjoyment of each other's company. Friends do not generally make demands of each other but when needed go beyond the call of duty. Supportive relationships enhance self-esteem and the sense of happiness and overall well-being and longevity. Conversely, loneliness and a lack of social supports have been linked to an increased risk of heart disease, infections and cancer, as well as higher mortality rates. Clinical trials document that lonely people don't recover as quickly from illness, don't sleep as well and develop high blood pressure. Philia or social interaction helps people be healthier and live longer.

Romantic love, or eros, has been celebrated throughout the ages and in all cultures. In classical mythology, Cupid, son of the love goddess Venus, is the god of desire and erotic love. In contemporary popular culture, Cupid with his bow and arrow lives on as the icon of Valentine's Day.

The Chinese celebrate the Qixi Festival. According to the legend, the Cowherd star and the Weaver Maid star, normally separated by the silvery river of the Milky Way are allowed to meet on this "lovers" day. In Brazil, single women perform rituals, called *sympatia*, on the *Dia dos Namorados* to find love.

The experience of "falling in love" is associated with three basic drives; liking or attraction (intimacy), the sex drive (lust or passion) and deep attachment (commitment).

Psychologist Robert Sternberg proposed a triangular theory in romantic love positing that the different combinations of the three components of love—intimacy, passion, and commitment—result in different types of love. For example, a combination of intimacy and commitment results in companionate love, while a combination of passion and intimacy leads to romantic love. Passion without intimacy or commitment is infatuation. Sex creates the illusion of union, but without intimacy or commitment this union remains physical, without depth. According to Sternberg, relationships built on two or more factors are more enduring than those based upon a single component. A combination of intimacy, passion and commitment is termed *consummate love*. This deepest and strongest form of love results in the greatest amount of dopamine release. This translates into lasting relationships with enduring satisfaction, health and happiness. Being in love improves immune functions and enhances health.

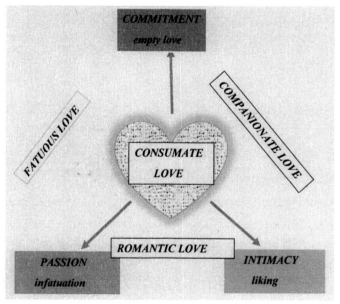

The initial attraction may be to a person's looks or movements or to their voice and enhanced by a person's adornments, clothing, and perfume. It is also influenced by psychological or cultural factors and personal standards.

The power of love to nurture and fulfill depends on commitment. A financial commitment should be spelt out early in the relationship with or without a prenuptial. Emotional commitment is a thoughtful and responsible decision to commit completely to the other. It requires a conscious choice for loyalty with a motivation to honor and trust the other. There is an unselfish vow to nurture and grow the other. It is to be vulnerable without humiliation or judgement. Commitment mandates sharing the burdens of daily chores and adversities as much as the joys and fun times.

Intimacy requires a sense of common goals and values, connecting at the level of the mind. There is a freedom of expression; to hear and be heard in return. It implies care, respect, and intimate knowledge of the other. There needs to be a willingness to be present to the other with integrity, allowing freedom to be oneself.

With passion, there is a thrill and pleasure in love making—a sense of urgency to be with the other.

In actuality, the person choosing to love determines the nature of the love. This love is exponentially enhanced by love that is reciprocated to the same degree.

In popular culture and through the media, the illusion of romantic love exists "till death do us part." In reality, falling in love is not uncommonly followed by heartbreak and disillusionment. It is an illusion that love means the absence of conflict. Conflicts approached with honesty and open communication can lead to a deeper knowledge of the other and strengthen the attachment.

True love is only possible if both communicate from the core or essence of one's being, caring for and growing the other.

Presumably to expand the gene pool, wild animals generally do not stick with one mate. There are a few exceptions, such as the penguins who wait for their mate every year during the mating season. In humans, monogamy makes for a more stable, social structure and a more supportive and nurturing environment, for self and offspring. Love grows deeper with time and shared experiences. It is also easy to take each other for granted and let familiarity and routines bury passion.

Knowing that there is not an in-built drive to stay with a single partner means having to work towards a lasting relationship. Our higher functioning neocortex (unlike animals) gives us the motivation and tools to make this choice. The seed of relationships need to be continually watered and fed to bear fruit —the fruit of physical, emotional and mental well-being.

Medical Applications

Knowing that positive neurochemicals are activated with the expression of love, reconnect with family and friends. Take time to grow and nurture love. Consider having a pet that you can love. Love gives a "high" that is more healthy than drugs or medications.

When we play the victim, or hold on to hurts, recounting what people did to us or did not do for us, we block the natural flow of love. Anxiety and depression is the end result. As in Rumi's poem about the elephant in the dark, each blind monk by their feel, perceived and described a part of the animal that differed from the others. The whole animal cannot be appreciated by a hand. Our perceptions are limited at best and we seldom know the whole story. We need to be tolerant of others whose thinking has led them to think and behave differently. Releasing past hurts and reconnecting with love is an act for liberation and peace.

Meditative Exercise

Find a quiet space and get comfortable. Start with the gentle abdominal breathing as before. Deepen the breath with slightly longer exhalations. Reminisce on the loves that you have experienced over the years. Love is always everywhere around you and within you. Only you can open your heart to love.

Bring to your mind's eye a person you love. Contemplate on what is lovable about him/her. Feel the essence of your loved one. Feel your heart swell as love and tenderness rush in. Let your love be as strong and unshakeable as a rock. Let this love spread to members in your family and then to a person that you have had a conflict with. Wish happiness and health for him/her. Then spread this love to all mankind and sentient beings.

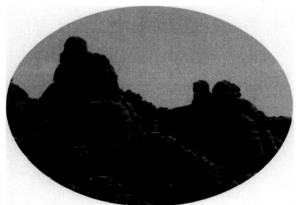

Monserrat, Spain

Be very still and let your thoughts go. Experience the mind-shift that occurs with the stillness.

CHAKRA 4

THE HEART CHAKRA
TWELVE PETALS OF VIRTUES

Agape & Altruism

Confidence & Courage

Equanimity & Empathy

Gratitude & Generosity

Humor & Humility

Patience & Perseverance

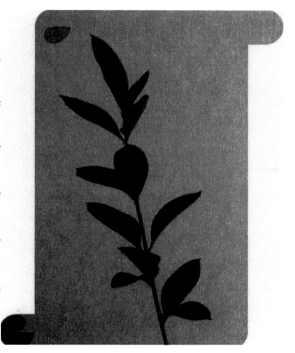

Chapter 18
TWELVE PETALS OF THE VIRTUES

"The line dividing good and evil cuts through the heart of every human being and who is willing to destroy a piece of his heart."
—Alexandr Solzhenitsyn, *The Gulag Archipelago*

The first three chakras are seen in all sentient beings in varying degrees and correlate to the reptilian brain and/or the mammalian brain. The fourth chakra or heart chakra involves the higher neocortex of humans. The fourth chakra is located at the level of the heart. The heart is traditionally said to be the seat of passion and the organ of life. For my purpose this is the chakra of the virtues. Virtue is a quality or a state of being rather than an emotion.

The Greek philosopher Aristotle (384—322 BCE) in his *Nicomachean Ethics*, outlines an ideal ethical model or framework within which humans deliberate and choose their actions in accordance with their moral virtues. His view entails a morally good, pleasurable and contemplative life.

A virtue involves reasoning that guides our actions; and when it is internalized, becomes an enduring character trait. It involves striving for excellence; in being human for the good of self and all. It is a "top down and out" activity that involves memory, executive functions, emotional expression, and language skills. These specific areas of the prefrontal cortex with their myriad connections to emotions and motor/sensory systems orchestrate the activity. In so doing pleasure hormones are released to produce a "feel-good" state. Rene Descartes says, *"Seek the sovereign good, as this produces a solid blessedness or pleasure."* Virtue represents the potential to live more fully and is a source of one's own wellbeing.

The online dictionary defines virtue as *"conformity of one's life and conduct to moral and ethical principles; the quality or practice of moral excellence or righteousness."* It is difficult to pinpoint an exact definition of virtues, but it is inextricably woven into morals, ethics and principles. Wikipedia defines morals as a personal, internal compass for right living. Ethics refers to rules of conduct, and principles as a code of conduct. Virtue is by choice, a mature, personal and moral orientation to life.

Aristotle defines virtue as a predisposition to behave in the right manner and is a mean between extremes of deficiency and excess, which are vices. According to Aristotle the goodness of any virtue is inseparable from the outcome of that virtue. If a virtuous trait were to lead to evil, it would not be a virtue at all, but rather a vice. In his *Nicomachean Ethics*, he states, *"At the right times, about the right things, towards the right people, for the right end, and in the right way, is the intermediate and best condition, and this is proper to virtue."* The point of greatest virtue lies at the mean sometimes closer to one extreme than the other. The yin/yang symbol expresses this concept well; the dividing line is a soft flowing S-like shape. As one aspect increases the other decreases. The mean moves to the right or left of center following the S-curve depending on the circumstances. Mean consists of finding an appropriate

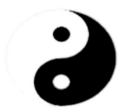

middle ground between two extremes which often is an exercise in judgment. As such, each virtue has two opposites. Thus the opposite of courage is both cowardice and recklessness; generosity fits between the two extremes of miserliness and extravagance. Wisdom is applying the right virtue in the right amount at the right time. There are four processes critical to virtuous behavior: awareness of the situation, discernment, motivation for good, followed by ethical action.

In Hindu philosophy, virtue is defined as something that cannot be imposed; it is something that is realized and voluntarily lived up to by each individual. It demands *careful and sustained reflection by every man and woman before it can become part of one's life* (Wikipedia). The Chinese philosopher Lao Tzu, author of the Tao Te Ching (book of the Way and its Virtue) 2,500 years ago chose the word "Tao" as the "Way" or natural order/wisdom of life. "Te" is translated as virtue or moral force. His teachings expand on virtues such as courage to face reality, the perseverance to solve problems and tranquility of mind to accept the outcome.

Virtually all cultures have a code of moral values. The Jews had their ten commandments written on stone brought down by Moses from the mountain top. Some of these codes were in the form of a negative "thou shalt not." The Samurai code is typified by seven virtues such as honor, respect and loyalty. Buddhism has the four "divine states" or virtues which are compassion, loving-kindness, altruism and equanimity. The ancient Hindu texts of the Vedas and Upanishads lists ten virtues to lead a life following the *natural laws* of *the universe*. The Lakota Indians lists twelve Lakota virtues. More recently, Peterson and Seligman developed a list of character strengths and virtues which they classified into six broad areas. These virtues showed similarity across cultures irrespective of race or religion. These six categories of virtue are courage, justice, humanity, temperance, transcendence, and wisdom. For my purpose, I list twelve virtues to represent the twelve petals of the fourth chakra:

1&2. Agape and Altruism
3&4. Courage and Confidence
5&6. Empathy and Equanimity
7&8. Gratitude and Generosity
9&10. Humor and Humility
11&12. Perseverance and Patience

Rather than viewing the virtues as isolated traits, a holistic view recognizes the interrelationships of the virtues with one another. It is when one is strong and stable at the core (state of equanimity) that one can give off oneself in empathy. It is with gratitude that one can be generous. And in persevering one learns patience.

Unfortunately, with industrialization, these virtues have become adulterated by economic values with the mean shifting towards vice. In general, however, we can have faith in the innate goodness of man, and most people would help rather than harm another. Though negative traits are present in human beings, the world is a compassionate place. Being raised in an atmosphere of moral merit motivates the development of these traits. Establishing proper virtues in children from a young age makes for moral excellence in the adult.

Our brains never lose the ability to learn by forming new connections and new cells. We can learn to develop positive qualities no matter how old we are. The more often a nerve pathway is used the greater the chance of it being fired, and fired faster. The neural pathways become stronger with repetition and the likelihood of use is increased. This has been proven with neuroimaging studies as the myelin sheath becomes thicker with use. The myelin sheath is the insulating protein and fatty membrane surrounding the nerve fibers. A thicker sheath allows a more rapid transmission of electrical information. The only way to become more virtuous is through practice. Through repetition, more of the 'feel-good' hormones are released and the sense of happiness increases.

Fowers (2005) defined virtues as character strengths that allow individuals to pursue their goals and ideals and to flourish as human beings. By actively pursuing virtues one could conceivably achieve eudemonia, which is defined as the fulfillment of one's potential for excellence and an enduring joy that flows from living a good life.

Green is the color that the heart chakra is associated with. Green is a secondary color and a meld of yellow and blue. In ancient Egyptian wall paintings, the ruler of the underworld, Osiris was typically portrayed with a green face, indicating his power to encourage growth. Egyptians honored the cycle of growth and decay and therefore green was also associated with death and resurrection. Green is the color of grass and leaves and associated with springtime, growth and nature. The green movement is allied with sustainability, and with being environmentally friendly. Green is the symbol of good health and rebirth. The virtues are environmentally friendly qualities. Nurturing these positive virtues sustains all life, fosters societal harmony and leads to increased individual happiness and wellness when practiced. The following chapters expand on a few of the virtues.

Chapter 19
AGAPE AND ALTRUISM

"I slept and I dreamed that life is all joy. I woke and I saw that life is all service. I served and I saw that service is joy."

—Kahlil Gibran

Agape love is the purest form of love and taken by religions to mean God's love or reciprocally the love of man for God. But in its true meaning it is unconditional, all-encompassing love. It is a "state of being" conforming to the supreme of virtues. It is a state embodied in the life of Christ as depicted in the bible. It is a state of "being love" —love emanating for all, unconditionally, with joy and understanding. Agape and altruism are the highest of ideals and not easy to live up to, continuously or consistently. However, we can hold these values as desirable goals and live up to them to the best of our ability during our lifespan.

In Christian theology agape love is referred to as charity. According to Thomas Aquinas, charity is an absolute requirement for happiness, which he holds as man's last goal. Chinese philosopher, Maze, stressed that love should be unconditional and offered to everyone without regard to reciprocation, and is a key element towards enlightenment. In Buddhist tradition agape love translates to 'metta', or loving-kindness, i.e. a caring for the happiness and well-being of another without expecting anything in return.

Agape love is a unique kind of love, a love devoid of sentimentality yet considerably more than kindness. A love based not on feelings but on the will. The reward is a sense of fulfillment, joy and positive feelings.

Agape love includes the quality of giving—whether it is talents, time and/or material goods, without reciprocation or reward. C. S. Lewis describes this as a selfless love committed to the well-being of the other. Agape therefore involves thought, effort, choice, and often self-sacrifice and self-denial.

One of the core commandments of Judaism and Christianity is *"Love thy neighbor as thyself* (Matthew 22:38 kjv)." In order to be able to truly love another person, one needs first to learn to love oneself. Paradoxically, love for self is intricately woven with love for others.

Loving oneself means caring about, taking responsibility for, respecting and knowing oneself (i.e. being realistic and honest about one's strengths and weaknesses). It is by loving oneself with *"true humility, courage, faith and discipline"* that one attains the capacity to experience real love.

Agape love involves stepping out of our own needs to become aware of and fulfill the needs of others. This act translates to altruism. Altruism is defined as practice of selfless concern for the well-being of others. We are generally programmed to take care of ourselves and to seek our own welfare and advantage. As humans, we have the ability to forego our own satisfactions for someone or something else if and when we choose.

In the mid to late twentieth century, many bought into Ayn Rand's philosophy. According to Ayn Rand, it is by living the morality of self-interest that one survives, flourishes, and achieves happiness. Rand, white-washes one's social conscience by rationalizing economic and social sins. Rand's philosophy argues that there is no social or moral obligation for one to help another; even if all others less fortunate in society (the poor, the sick, the disabled,) are left to fend for themselves and suffer and die.

Rand's extremist views probably emerged because her family lost everything when their property was confiscated by the Bolshevik Party under Vladimir Lenin during the Bolshevik Revolution in 1917. Probably her negative experience with extreme Marxist socialism, led her to propound her views of capitalism and pure self-interest. Her view of a life of sacrificing others for one's own end has shaped history and contributed to the recent economic collapse. The resulting bankruptcy, banking collapse and high unemployment clearly shows the perils of this selfish route. The misconception of the catchphrase "the selfish gene," (related to evolutionary concepts and not human behavior) promoted by Richard Dawkins probably compounded matters.

The other extreme view of a life of sacrificing one's own end for others led to socialist utopian communities with the ideal of people working and living together with equal rights. These communities required personal sacrifices for the "common good" of all. The intent was to replace a system of selfish competition with brotherly cooperation. These utopian communities failed for the most part; as human traits, aspirations and abilities are so diverse, that demanding equality of cooperation, sacrifice and effort is unrealistic. The weaknesses of extreme capitalism or socialism articulate the wisdom of the "Aristotelian mean" for an effective society.

We do not know exactly where altruism of humans come from. But it appears to stem from tribal identification. We must cooperate in order to survive, and we are altruistic to others because we need them for our survival. Humans developed cooperative skills because it was in their mutual interest to work well with others. It began in small hunter-gatherer groups and has become more complex and culturally engraved in modern societies.

Selfless love is tied in with justice. Working for the good of all, benefits society as a whole and ultimately self as well. Individual acts of altruism can have far reaching effects. Suffrage, civil rights, social security and entitlements would not have come about without those that cared deeply about social good.

Being altruistic and kind to one another benefits all. In this current global environment, it is imperative that communities appreciate the significance and importance of agape love and altruism, and express it as a lived reality with mutual cooperation, interdependence and social responsibility.

Being selfless and giving, opens us to the risk of rejection, hurt and betrayal. It can lead to feelings of resentment or we might feel that we are being taken advantage of or undervalued. Being over-taxed by the needs of others we can 'burn out' with negative effects on health and happiness. Selfless love, empathy and altruism involve internal struggles. Ultimately, people are responsible for their own welfare, which helps us find equanimity in the face of other's suffering. It is only by developing a core of self-sufficiency, equanimity, strength, and clarity of purpose that we can be more likely to engage in altruistic activities with authenticity. A tendency toward altruistic behavior probably develops through learning and exposure to appropriate social practices during childhood or adolescence when the brain is rapidly developing. However, the brain maintains plasticity and can be molded as an adult.

Researchers have found a strong association between altruistic behavior and the volume of gray matter in an area of the brain known as the temporo-parietal junction (TPJ) involved in appreciating others' perspectives. Individuals who work at understanding others' intents and beliefs are more altruistic than those who do not care. It has also been found that the amygdala was significantly larger and super-sensitive in altruists and blunted in psychopaths, who are unresponsive to the feelings of others.

Making time to be of service to others provides joy that is deeply renewing. By caring and connectedness, our own deepest needs are satisfied.

Medical Applications

Agape and altruistic behavior are intertwined with happiness. The giving and receiving of altruistic love increases personal well-being and health. A loving body absorbs less cholesterol, increases the production of immunoglobulins and beneficial hormones, such as DHEA which is antiaging. Cultivating unconditional loving-kindness reduces anger and hostility, boosts positive emotions and improves sleep. Serving the needs of others with caring and selflessness leads to joy and satisfaction, fulfilling our unspoken innermost needs. Looking for good in others starts the flow of positive synchrony. Healing is about engaging and being present with the experience.

Loving-kindness meditation has been shown to lower stress and inflammation, both of which are associated with major depression, heart disease and diabetes. Inflammation also increases the risk of Alzheimer's dementia.

"A change of heart changes everything" is the slogan for the "Heart Math" team. Research done by this team of medical scientists showed that patterns in the heart rhythm corresponds to specific emotional states. Feelings of love and compassion leads to a coherent (harmonious) heart rhythm that in turn leads to other positive chemical and neurological reactions in the body. The synchronization of heart and mind translates to an internal radiance. According to ancient Hasidic Jews, *"wear nothing around the neck to block the connection between brain and heart."*

By understanding neurobiology, behavioral and cognitive therapies can be developed to compensate for deficits in social functions in patients with autism and other forms of neuropsychiatric illness. Future research evaluating the cellular and molecular mechanisms underlying these complex social functions can help pave the way for pharmacological treatments.

Meditative Exercise

Knowing that selfless love leads to personal gratification and happiness, adopt a pet or engage in volunteer activities. Small attempts such as picking up litter in your neighborhood or taking food in to an elderly can lead to large gains in personal happiness.

The Buddhist practice of loving-kindness meditation involves sending metta (loving kindness and goodwill) to oneself, to a close person, then an adversary and the universe in turn.

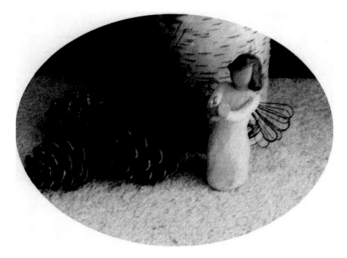

Loving kindness meditation can be practiced in any posture such as reclining, sitting, standing and walking. It is best to do what works for you.

Spend a few minutes relaxing any tight spots as tension can be a distraction and obstacle to loving kindness. Gently stretch your arms overhead followed by gentle rotations of the neck. Breathe a garden of peace to surround you. Let go of distractions and thoughts about the day. Being kind to yourself in this way can prepare the mind to relax and be more open to the practice.

Bathe yourself in loving-kindness, letting go of self-criticism. We can offer love to others only if we can claim it for ourselves. If a distraction or a resentful thought arises, observe the feeling and the stress of such a thought. Let go of the thought and return to your focus with the wish "May I be love…... May I be tolerant and free of judgment."

Explore the needs and feelings of a loved one followed by a conscious intention to be of service. In the same way, consider the needs and feelings for someone with whom you are in conflict. Then expand this wish to all sentient beings in turn. Be present with the experience of expansive love spilling and radiating out while opening your heart and mind to the service of others.

Let negative thoughts go as they arise, or use them as a basis of understanding. Observe the way ill-will or negative thoughts can overpower goodwill or positive thoughts.

In all our relationships, whether family, friends, acquaintances, co-workers and lovers, this meditation can help us gain more patience and *insight* into our interactions, and help us take positive steps towards authentic agape and altruism. Develop equanimity by stepping back with detached observation and inner balance.

Engage in this practice in the evenings; awake to the morning, energized by love and a renewed commitment to a life of service balanced by self-care.

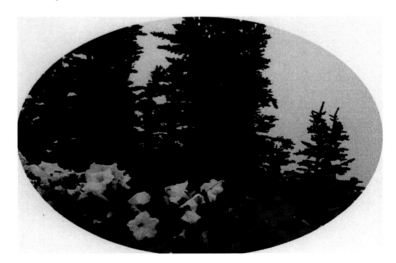

Crystal Mountain, Washington

Chapter 20
CONFIDENCE AND COURAGE

"It's not the size of the dog in the fight, it's the size of the fight in the dog."
—Mark Twain

"Physical bravery is an animal instinct; moral bravery is much higher and truer courage."
—Wendell Phillips

Confidence is a virtue that conforms to Aristotle's mean. The extreme on the spectrum being pride or hubris and at the other end, timidity or low self-esteem. Self-confidence is the essential enabler in one's life. Confidence allows us to acknowledge doubts and yet permits us to persist and overcome, trusting that things will work out. A doubt becomes a challenge rather than a paralysis by all the "what ifs." Confidence is believing that we have what it takes to handle whatever happens and not let fear, doubt or worry stop us.

Low self-confidence or self-esteem impacts all of us at different points in our lives. Lacking faith in our abilities, our attractiveness, or our relationship skills is a common theme in the human drama. These difficulties and challenges may be problems we've faced since childhood. Self-confidence isn't developed by escaping these difficulties, but rather it's nurtured and strengthened by the way we respond to these circumstances and how we view ourselves in spite of them.

Confidence does not mean that we can achieve anything or think that we are the best. It does not mean we feel no anxiety or are invincible. Confidence is about embracing your inherent worth and your ability to accept and live with your successes and failures and not let the problems in your life stop you from trying again.

> *"Confidence comes not from always being right but from not fearing to be wrong."*
> —Peter T. McIntyre

It is about having a determined attitude of being able to overcome the next time around. Self-confidence is about taking a risk and carrying on in spite of. Confidence means that you try and try again. It is what turns thoughts into actions. With action comes more confidence. Small changes and tiny steps, can make a difference. Perseverance and patience pays off. With each successful experience comes growth of self-confidence. Confidence, in turn, is what leads to the courage to act.

Wikipedia defines courage as *the ability and willingness to confront fear, pain, danger, uncertainty, or intimidation.* Courage is the quality of mind that enables a person to face adversity and come through.

Legendary heroes famous for acts of courage are immortalized in myths and folk tales. Heracles in Greek mythology is born to mortal parents and begins exhibiting feats of great strength and bravery as a baby. Perseus, boldly marches to behead the Gorgon *Medusa*, and saves Andromeda from the sea monster Cetus. In the old testament of the Hebrew Bible, David faces the giant Goliath and defeats him with nothing but a puny sling. Hollywood's superheroes and action heroes continue the heroic and inspirational tales of Superman and Luke Skywalker in Star Wars. The hero goes out to face trials and ordeals, and comes back victorious. History books tell colorful tales of social activists, such as Martin Luther King and Nelson Mandela, who chose to speak out against injustice at great personal risk.

From the perspective of Buddhism, courage is the quality that enables us to expand our lives and manifest our inner potential to do the difficult thing we know to be right, to be empowered and not overpowered by fear or apathy. *"Courage is …the mastery of fear—not absence of fear,"* writes Mark Twain in the novel *Pudd'nhead Wilson*.

Just as every part of the human body has a function so also every part of the human brain has specific functions. Courageous acts seem to activate a part of the prefrontal cortex called the anterior cingulate cortex (ACC). The ACC acts as an important interface between emotion and cognition, converting feelings into actions. This area is involved in executive functions such as the control of one's emotions, problems solving, and adapting to changing conditions. The amygdala, where the fear is triggered, is close to and also connected to the ACC. A strongly active ACC overrides the physiological and psychological response to fear driven by the amygdala, and allows people to act courageously. The prefrontal cortex allows for the mastery of fear. This account is probably an oversimplified explanation in the whole dynamics of courage as many other executive functions in the frontal cortex are involved and called into play.

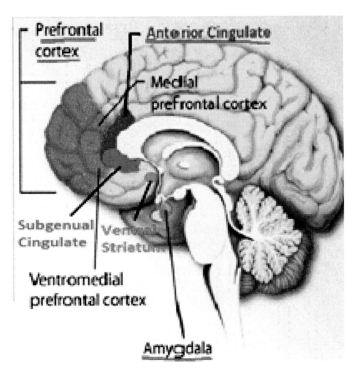

ANTERIOR CINGULATE CORTEX
Mmm Daffodils via Wikimedia commons

We do not have to be a hero to exhibit courage. There are many possibilities each day to act courageously. Sometimes it is just the sheer determination at the end of the day to try again and do better tomorrow. Sisyphus was condemned to roll a boulder up the side of a mountain over and over again for eternity, but yet had an attitude of fortitude. The boulder represents the not so glamorous aspects of daily living with and among others.

It takes a gentle sort of courage to face the grind of daily living. It takes courage to say 'no' as well as to say 'yes' when indicated. It takes courage to admit when we are mistaken, ignorant or have trouble understanding; to stand by our beliefs and for what we know is right; to dream and move out of our comfort zone.

> *"It takes courage ... to endure the sharp pains of self-discovery rather than choose to take the dull pain of unconsciousness that would last the rest of our lives."*
> —Marianne Williamson,
> *A Return to Love*

Courage does not lie in drugs or alcohol but in nurturing our belief that we can overcome situations and come out whole.

Medical Applications

Soldiers in spite of going through brave courageous acts in war are torn with a myriad of postwar mental and emotional diagnoses. This is partly related to the mismatch between the courageous act and the values they hold. The values of human dignity, respect, and agape love and altruism are violated when one has to kill and destroy.

With the scientific discoveries and the role of the anterior cingulate cortex, medications can be developed to target this area and lead to innovative ways to deal with fear based diagnoses such as panic attacks and phobias.

Meditative Exercise

Be inspired by the courage and confidence of the tiniest of birds, the hummingbirds, as they make their solitary migrations between Central America and North America/Canada. These migratory journeys span hundreds or thousands of miles at an average rate of about twenty miles per day, advancing and retreating with the seasons to claim the best feeding places in conjunction with flowering time.

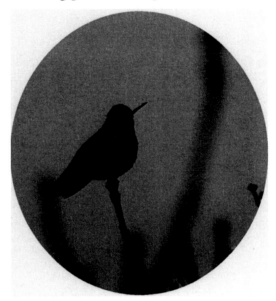

Durga is the Hindu goddess of courage. Her creation was the result of the many gods held captive by the evil Mahisa. The gods gave her ten arms and weapons to fend off the fearsome Mahisa. These multiple arms offered protection from all corners of the earth. With this unsurpassed power Durga freed the gods. Durga reminds us that we have the many arms of our friends and family to equip us with the tools we need to courageously embark on our journey of life with confidence.

Set aside a time to relax in your favorite spot, away from the busyness of life. It may be in a quiet corner of your home or somewhere in nature. Take time to reflect on the many hands that have held you through life's path. The hands that held you as you took your first step as a toddler. The hands that led you through first grade and beyond. Reflect on the risks taken and the successes experienced throughout your life. With each step, self-worth and confidence have grown and the courage to step beyond is greater. You are amassing tools to go further on a daily basis. You continue to bloom and grow.

Gently close your eyes and let your breathing be even and regulated. Center and calm the mind. Give thanks for the many arms of your family and friends embracing and encircling you. Close with a simple affirmation of: "I appreciate my family and friends who support and encourage me. I am worthy. I have achieved. I have the courage to face life with confidence. I have the courage to let go of past hurts and welcome new possibilities. I can be more."

Chapter 21
GRATITUDE AND GENEROSITY

"You give but little when you give of your possessions. It is when you give of yourself that you truly give."
—Khalil Gibran, *The Prophet*

"Be the flower that gives its fragrance to even the hand that crushes it"

—Ali ibn Abi Talib

From the earliest times man has had a need to express gratitude to the unknown giver of food, water and air. This sense of indebtedness gave rise to sacrificial acts dating at least as far back as 1200 BCE.

Human sacrifice was considered the highest in repayment of debt, a symbol of life returned for the life enjoyed. According to the Old Testament, Abraham was ready to sacrifice his own son. The Israelites offered a young sheep and first fare from the harvest as commemoration and atonement. The sacrifice generally was central to the belief that it was an offering on behalf of all.

This belief is carried on to this day in the Christian belief of Jesus as sacrifice for the sins of the world.

Gratitude for the fruit of the land is seen as harvest celebrations. In Egypt the spring-time harvest festival was dedicated to Min, their god of vegetation and fertility. Israel celebrates Sukkot (feast of the ingathering) with sheaves of willow, myrtle, date palm fronds and citron that represent the blessings of nature. In Bali small dolls of rice stalks dedicated to Dewi Sri the rice goddess, are placed in granaries as offerings. The Roman celebration of Cerelia, a harvest festival, is dedicated to Ceres, their goddess of corn. Kwanzaa originated from African harvest festivals and celebrates the first fruits of harvest. Lighting candles, reciting prayers, singing songs and giving gifts are rituals of thanksgiving seen in virtually all cultures.

Multiple measures or scales of gratitude have been devised to measure and define gratitude, e.g. Adler and Fagley's *Appreciation Scale*. Basically, gratitude is to notice and acknowledge the value and meaning of what we have, what we have received, what we experience (even hardship), and of life itself. A factor in developing gratitude is acceptance. Acceptance of our circumstances leads to a lack of resentment for what we have or do not have. It is not difficult to express thanks for our material possessions or the helping hand extended when we needed it. But when we add reverence and awe to the feeling of appreciation, we transcend the feeling into a state of gratitude.

So many of life's simple pleasures are free and there for the taking if we bring awareness to it. Gratitude involves feeling reverence for what we often take for granted—the sun's warmth, a cool breeze on one's face and the soft green grass underfoot, and the magic of stars and rainbows.

Michael Josephson says that what the world needs more of, is people to appreciate and enjoy the beautiful mountains and lush forests, and the promise of a sunrise and sunset every day.

Gratitude is a virtue that imprints our emotions and thoughts, and translates into positive actions. *Acts of* generosity is one way we express that gratitude.

The French phrase "Noblesse oblige" originated from the implicit responsibility of the advantaged class to act with generosity and nobility toward those less privileged. On Boxing Day, the day after Christmas, in accordance with old English tradition, the wealthy gave their servants a box of leftover food from the Christmas feast, the day off, and other gifts.

Andrew Carnegie (1889) in *The Gospel of Wealth* proposed that the best way of dealing with wealth inequality was for the wealthy to reallocate their surplus wealth in a responsible and thoughtful manner to the worthy without encouraging idleness. Generosity should not be just a virtue of individuals but also a corporate responsibility, because ultimately, it is a high-return strategy, even though the potential for gain may not be immediately apparent.

As the Chinese proverb says, *"Give a man a fish, you feed him for a day. Teach a man to fish, you feed him for a lifetime."* Aristotle suggests giving to the right people, in the right amounts, at the right time, with pleasure, and without looking out for oneself. The attitude of the generous gesture being more important than the gift itself.

Emmanuel Levinas, however, maintains that true generosity does not discriminate between more or less deserving recipients.

All religious traditions, the Abrahamic traditions in particular, stress showing generous hospitality towards the stranger, offering shelter and food. A small act of generosity might make a world of difference to someone. Buddhism lists generosity as a quality for the path of perfection; the ultimate act of generosity being the giving of oneself rather than wealth or possessions. Sharing time, knowledge, talents and being emotionally available for someone in need is true generosity given with love and without expectations. Generosity allows us detachment from material things. A generous spirit overcomes intolerance and paves the way for love and forgiveness. *"It is the heart that does the giving; the fingers only let go,"* according to a Nigerian proverb.

Scientists have discovered that choosing generosity over selfishness, makes the brain light up with joy. There is a sense of pleasure for having done something good. It involves neurochemical changes in the brain with the release of the pleasure hormone, oxytocin. By donating money to a charity, the same neural network showed *greater* activity than receiving money. The joy of being a giver is a worthwhile investment, greater than that of being a recipient.

On the flip side, we need to be gracious in accepting help and gifts; but we should never be dependent on, or take advantage of the generosity of others.

Medical Applications

An attitude of gratitude has been shown to have a strong link with positive mental health and well-being. It correlates with higher levels of happiness and lower levels of anxiety, stress and depression. Research conducted at University of California found that gratitude gives the person expressing it a stronger immune system improving the power to heal, Sleep quality is improved and the body energized. Grateful people have higher levels of personal growth and purpose in life. They tend to be more compassionate and more optimistic, and have more positive ways of coping with the difficulties they experience in life.

People who are emotionally available and hospitable are much more likely to be in excellent health than those who are not.

Studies have found that the happier you are, the more likely you are to be generous. The more generous you are the more oxytocin is released, increasing the level of happiness.

Meditative Exercise
Each morning on awakening, cultivate gratitude and "awesomize" and not "awfulize."

Lay on your back in your comfortable bed. Let your hands relax by your side palms up. Let your eyes gently close. Relax the muscles around your forehead and eyes. Let your tongue rest on the upper palette releasing tension in the jaws. Breathe in slowly and gently starting from your feet and through your torso up to the crown. Exhale, letting the breath wash down the back and back out through the feet.

Take a moment to practice naming three awesome things you are grateful for. Pay attention to your heart as your mind recalls these things; be aware of the softening, the opening.

It's the perfect way to start the day right whether you are sad, angry or emotionally drained. Accept, with gratitude, that pain and difficult situations are part of life. With acceptance comes release and a step toward healing and wholeness.

As you go about your day be mindful of ways you can be generous. Share a smile or a kind word. Take time to be with another giving them your full attention. Be mindful of the graciousness of another toward you, accepting it with gratitude. Life is a series of give and take.

End the day reflecting on the generosity that you have experienced.

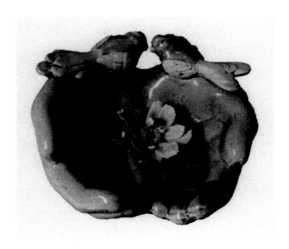

Chapter 22
HUMOR AND HUMILITY

"Laughter is the sun that drives winter away from the human face."

—Victor Hugo

"A sense of humor is just common sense dancing."
—William James.

Smiling emerges roughly five weeks after birth and laughter as early as two to four months old. Laughter is absolutely critical in establishing and maintaining social interactions across cultures. It has been determined that ten to fifteen minutes of laughter a day can burn up to forty calories. Hence laughter yoga was made popular as an exercise by Indian physician Madan Kataria. In the mid-1990s, laughter yoga was practiced in the early mornings in open parks, primarily by groups of older people. This movement has spread worldwide as "Laughter Clubs." Laughter facilitates laughter in others and improves social bonding. However this laughter is superficial and is akin to casual sex, i.e. superficial without depth of meaning.

Humor on the other hand is a deeper state of mind that involves seeing the absurdity in situations and how we react to things that happen to us or others.

Having a sense of humor isn't just connected to telling jokes or even being funny. Having a sense of humor is about having a sense of perspective about our day to day problems and challenges. It's about using our humor resources to keep equilibrium in a crisis, to manage stress and to problem-solve in a more creative fashion. Laughing in the face of a crisis helps us to face our problems head on. Learning to take ourselves lightly we develop the ability to rise above any situation. As with all other virtues, there is a negative side or dark side to humor that is hostile and manipulative. Cruel attacks based on race, sex, ethnicity, religion, or other aspects of people's identity is hurtful and contemptible as it tears communities and societies apart.

The perception of humor depends on numerous cognitive skills and extensive neurological networking with memory, abstract thinking, social perception, emotional expression and language. It's a mental ability that gets our emotions and our bodies involved in the act. The comical event is processed by the ventromedial prefrontal cortex, the anterior cingulate cortex, the amygdala, and the ventral striatum of the limbic system. These sites in turn, influence the hypothalamus, the cranial nerves and motor regions to generate the complex laughter reaction. The eyes wrinkle, mouth opens with corners turned up, a deep throated "Ha Ha" sound coordinates with respiration and contraction of the diaphragm. The belly ripples and shakes with the laughter. Occasionally we double up or fallover to roll on the floor. It is truly a positive mind-body collaboration.

In Greek mythology, the goddess Baubo is celebrated as a fun-loving, bawdy, sexually liberated force depicting the healing power of laughter. Medieval European courts employed court jesters who, taking advantage of their license to speak freely would use humor in the form of irony, exaggeration, or ridicule to expose and criticize people's stupidity or vices.

Kant describes the enjoyment of joking and wit as *"the play of thought."* To find things funny we need to be able to shift perspective, perceive incongruities and paradoxes, and be surprised and delighted by the unexpected punch line, the pun and play of words.

To enjoy humor one needs to be in the right frame of mind; boredom, anger or fear inhibits laughter.

Viktor Frankl, in his book, *Man's Search for Meaning*, recounts his experience surviving a holocaust camp during World War II. Frankl attributes his ability to rise up above his unspeakably horrific circumstances to his sense of humor. *"Humor was another of the soul's weapons in the fight for self-preservation,"* writes Frankl. He describes how his inner spirit, including his sense of humor, was the one thing no one could ever take away from him and he claims that humor helped save his life.

The ability to laugh at and not take ourselves seriously and to see the humor in our circumstances leads to humility.

Ralph Sockman describes true humility as *intelligent self-respect which keeps us from thinking too highly or too meanly of ourselves.*

Humility derives from the Latin *humus*, meaning earth or ground. The earth from which we came and where all must go keeps us grounded with humility.

Humility is defined as a modest view of one's own importance.

The extremes in the humility spectrum are pride on the one hand and self-effacement at the other. Humility requires us to value ourselves without pride or self-negation.

The mark of humility is recognizing and feeling oneness with everyone and everything else in the universe, without inferiority or superiority. It is the virtue of knowing our own limitations, our inadequacies and dependencies; the strength of admitting we're not always right; the knowledge that we are not infallible and that other people have something to teach us. The research suggests that humility is multi-dimensional involving multiple neural networks in the prefrontal cortex. It includes self-understanding and awareness, openness and perspective taking.

Eastern philosophical traditions understand humility as a process of self-emptying and self-forgetting; a rigorous discipline that involves a relentless training exemplified by the Tibetan monks. Humility is an elusive quality, as in the very act of striving to appear to be humble, we exhibit pride of our humility. Jesus pointed this out in his rebuke of those who ostentatiously fast or pray in public, to advertise their virtuousness.

Ancient societies with their stories and myths teach the danger of hubris and the importance of humility. Most of the world's religions value humility above other qualities. In the King James Bible, Jesus is quoted as saying *"Blessed are the meek: for they shall inherit the earth."* In Hinduism, humility is the non-judgmental state of mind when we are best able to learn, contemplate and understand everyone and everything else. Taoists value humility as one of the three treasures (virtues), compassion and frugality being the other two. According to Confucius, humility is the solid foundation of all virtues. Treating each person as someone of value irrespective of their position in society, profession, age or economic status, demonstrates great humility. Leadership with humility is understanding that we are nothing without those working with us. This model of leadership fosters loyalty.

Gandhi, an example of true humility said, *"It is unwise to be too sure of one's own wisdom. It is healthy to be reminded that the strongest might weaken and the wisest might err."* Harijan (1940). It is challenging to be humble in a society that fosters self-indulgence and places high value on material wealth. But the benefits which include peace, wisdom, healthier relationships and the respect of others are well worth the effort.

By catching ourselves bragging or valuing our opinions above others or becoming unduly preoccupied with appearances we develop more humility.

Medical Applications

It has been said that laughter is the best medicine. Scientific studies have indicated that laughter yoga may have some medically beneficial effects to cardiovascular health and mood. Hearty laughing improves respiratory function and cardiac output. A deep belly laugh oxygenates the blood, relaxes and stimulates the abdominal muscles, and improves heart rate and blood pressure. A study by the Oxford University found that laughter raised pain thresholds probably by an endorphin-mediated opiate effect. Laughing alleviates stress, reduces depression and anxiety. There is an adage that 'mirth' is like a flash of lightning that breaks through a cloud of gloom. A sense of humor lightens life's obstacles and troubles.

Humor can influence interpersonal relationships, easing tension and facilitating communication and plays a crucial role in social bonding and camaraderie. By experience we know that we feel better after a good hearty laugh. Humor and laughter can be integrated into a holistic wellness plan that can translate into improvements in mind, body, and spirit.

Meditative Exercise

Spend time with a young child and watch a cartoon together. Laugh heartily at the comic characters. Experience the feeling of wellness and exuberance that laughter brings. Enjoy the laughter of your young companion. Notice how your laughter reinforces his/hers and how the child's laughter in turn stimulates yours.

Take time to be quiet in your favorite spot. Let your breath be even and flowing like a gentle river. Let your breath be long, slow inhalations and long, slow exhalations. Be mindful of all the sensations in your body without allowing them to interrupt your breath. Let your thoughts settle like pebbles in a pond, leaving it open, calm and clear.

Reflect on your most significant achievements. Recall the circumstances and the people involved to make this happen. Realize that success cannot happen in a vacuum. No success happens by one's own endeavor. Accept with humility all the skills and capabilities you have been blessed with. Reflect with humility on the nature of interdependence. The mountains, water and temperatures fashion the scenic beauty. The glaciers will be nonexistent without the right conditions.

Let your mind drift back to your breath with new awareness and appreciation.

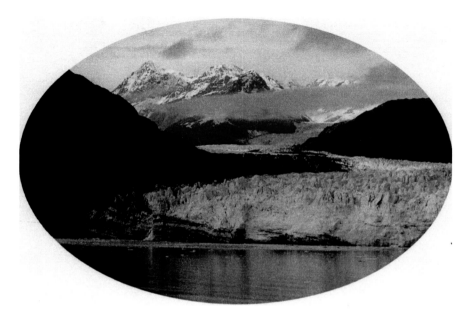

Glacier Bay, Alaska

CHAKRA 5
THROAT CHAKRA
SIXTEEN PETALS OF EXPRESSION

HISTORY

Culture

Beliefs

Memory

Ego

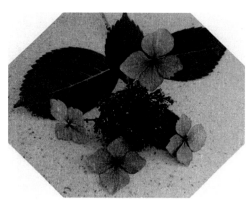

EXTRINSIC

Language

Knowledge

Skills

Vocation

INTRINSIC

Genetics

Temperament

Intellect

Conscience

POTENTIAL

Imagination

Creativity

Will

Choice

Chapter 23
SIXTEEN PETALS OF EXPRESSION

*"Wise men speak because they have something to say;
Fools because they have to say something."*

—Plato

*"Your living is determined not so much by what life
brings to you as by the attitude you bring to life; not so
much by what happens to you as by the way your mind
looks at what happens."*

—Khalil Gibran

The fifth Chakra or the throat chakra is located at the level of
the throat and is the seat of expression—the expression of self
as an individual. It is an expression or manifestation of oneself
and is the totality of one's self construct. The health factor of
the fifth chakra is in relation to how honestly we express ourselves. It directly reflects our willingness to be true to ourselves
without losing sight of the thoughts, understandings and con-
cerns of those around us. We were generally brought up with

the adage "Children should be seen and not heard." The intent was to cause us to learn to speak and act in socially acceptable ways. As we mature we exert our choices regarding behavior and manner.

The Greek god, Hermes, personifies this chakra with his power of speech and eloquence as well as his creativity and innovation. He is the herald and messenger of the gods and the promoter of social dialogue. Being creative he is said to have invented the alphabet and numbers, measures and weights, astronomy, music and the cultivation of the olive tree.

We can identify with the throat chakra when we experience that "lump in our throat" when we are at a loss to say the right words in a sticky situation. Expression can be in the form of verbal communication or it can be an artistic rendering, as in an artist's painting, a dancer's dancing, a musician's recital or any other form for expressing and bringing to the outside what was within. In my chakra interpretation, expression is uniquely individual and is a process of projecting oneself outwards, expressing oneself in speech, manner, behavior, and performance. Renowned photographer Ansel Adams has said that no man has the right to dictate what other men should perceive, create or produce; and that everyone should be encouraged to reveal themselves, their perceptions and emotions.

The chakras, as stated in earlier chapters, are depicted as vortices of energy. The vortex concept is beautifully illustrated in this chakra. The different components that make up this chakra are interrelated; growing and changing with time like a spiraling tornado. As a child our experience and knowledge is limited. As we grow, our field of abilities and knowledge expands in ever enlarging spirals. Each twist building up from what went before and expanding outwards with the next. Or it can be likened to the unfolding of a flower in time-lapse. Each petal as it unfurls is perfect and beautiful but the whole flower is more than the sum of the petals.

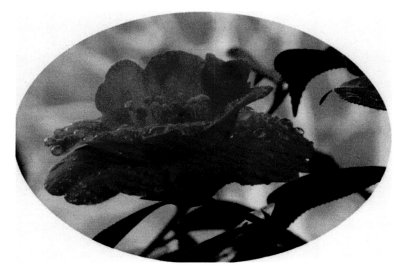

The factors of the fifth chakra are influenced by the most developed part of the brain known as the cortex. The cortex or the rind of the cerebral hemispheres is known as the grey matter and is made up of nerve cells. The most sophisticated and highly developed part of the cortex is the frontal lobe. This is the executive chamber zoned for decision making, planning, memory and personality.

These functions are carried out by a cascade of communications through neural networks or nerve fibers that are protected by a fatty myelin sheath (the white matter). Our knowledge of computer networks offers us a glimpse into the complexity of neural networks in the brain.

Sherrington describes the brain as an enhanced loom where millions of flashing shuttles weave meaningful patterns. These changeable patterns reflect the brain's ability to form new nerve connections throughout life—a quality referred to as neuroplasticity. Neuroplasticity allows neurons (nerve cells) in the brain to heal and compensate when injured.

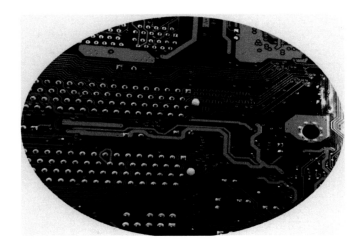

In the embryonic brain there is an excess of nerve cells and synapses which over time is shaped and pruned by the environment and interpersonal interactions. Cells that are not used or needed, die and are eliminated. New cell formation (neurogenesis) from stem cells in the brain and new synaptic connections (synaptogenesis) continues to occur throughout life. It is estimated that adult human brains have 100 billion neurons or nerve cells. These nerve cells have 10,000 connections to other neurons creating two million miles of neural tracts! This is absolutely mind-boggling, considering the human brain occupies the space of two hands held side by side. *"The brain is wider than the sky,"* the concept beautifully captured by Emily Dickinson.

The activity of our billions of neurons is the critical feature of our mental world. Functional magnetic resonance imaging (fMRI) has allowed us to map the brain and understand the role of each brain region and how they are zoned to collaborate and support mental functions. Different areas of the cerebral cortex have specialized functions; synapses and circuits integrate the whole into a harmonious, incredibly complex system. As we experience and learn, we form new synaptic connections. Repetitive stimulation and interaction strengthens the myelin fibers and the neural circuit, much as repetitive travel over a dirt road forms well-worn ruts. Experience significantly affects the shaping, sculpting and pruning of the brain. As neurons develop and connections form, our perception of the world becomes more integrated. We fill in sensory incoming data or interpret a sequence of events with existing internal data or prior information to form new perceptions.

The brain processes everything that we are exposed to. It is a dynamic structure sculpted through use throughout life. The more we know about one area, the more significant the other areas seem to become in explaining the whole picture. The mind pieces together incoming data to make sense of our complex world and create a coherent picture. But what we think and perceive about the world is a "second hand story" and not always the truth and neither does it always reflect what another brain thinks.

Paradoxically, the more we learn about the mind the more we realize that we can never reduce human thought, feeling, or behavior to a biochemical or electrical activity. Little known mechanisms for intuition and synchronicity play a part in our daily interactions.

The color of the fifth chakra is blue, a primary color. It's nature's color for sky and ocean and associates with expansive horizons. Dust particles in the sky absorb all the colors in the sky except blue which has the fastest vibration. This blue color of the sky is reflected back in the waters of the sea.

Experiments with undergraduates and color show that being exposed to blue stimulates the creative process. Surveys in the United States and Europe show that blue is the most popular color, chosen by almost half of both men and women as their favorite. It is associated with harmony, infinity, the imagination, and conveys a sense of trust, loyalty and cleanliness. Blue is the color used for the clothing of the Virgin Mary and became associated with holiness, humility, and virtue. In the United States, the blue ribbon is usually the highest award in expositions and county fairs. 'Blue' is used in American cultural expression as in "singing the blues" and "feeling blue."

The artist Yves Klein describes blue as the invisible being made visible. The factors that are instrumental in the expression of our abstract invisible nature of self can be illustrated using the acronym BLUE.

B is for beyond and represents factors that are yet to be manifest or one's potentialities. These potentialities or as yet un-manifested characteristics to grow and develop are governed by the imagination, creativity, choice and intent or will.

L is for lemons.

"When life gives you lemons—make lemonade"
—Elbert Hubbard.

Lemons are the intrinsic and inherent characteristics that life hands us. These factors include our genetics, temperament, intellect and conscience. Lemons are not necessarily bad and we do not inevitably need to stay stuck in what life gave us. We can change these factors and make lemonade or lemon meringue pie.

U is for the underlying or past experiences that influence and govern our lives. It is the history of what went before but yet influences the present and the future. It involves culture, beliefs, memory and ego.

E is for the extrinsic factors that knead and shape us. It is the load on the camel that Nietzsche describes in the three transformations of the spirit. It involves receiving instruction and information in order to live a responsible life in the society. This includes language, knowledge, skills, and vocation.

Thus the four categories of our unrealized potential, the intrinsic factors, our past experiences or history and the extrinsic factors, each with its four subcategories make up the sixteen petals of the fifth chakra to be expanded upon in the following chapters.

Chapter 24
THE INTRINSICS

"Labor to keep alive in your breast that little spark of celestial fire called conscience."

—George Washington,
Rules of Civility And Other Writings

"Let us understand what our own selfish genes are up to. Because we may then at least have the chance to upset their designs."

—Richard Dawkins

Genetics, temperament, intellect and conscience, modulated by a host of factors, are the intrinsic, dynamic elements whereby we express ourselves.

Our human genes came from single celled organisms that through evolutionary pathways evolved to bacteria, plants, lower animals and humans. Inside the nucleus of a cell, our genes are arranged along molecules of DNA called chromosomes.

The nucleus of every cell in the human body contains twenty-three pairs of chromosomes that hold the code for and are responsible for heredity. Each chromosome is made up of DNA, a twisted, double-stranded chemical spiral made up of smaller molecules. Genes are made of "bits" of three-dimensional protein codes which are small areas on these spirals that transmit the instruction for a particular process or characteristic. Some characteristics are the result of a single gene but more commonly many genes work together in its expression.

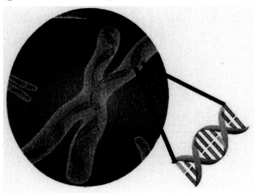

Researchers have unraveled the human genome (total gene make-up). We possess about thirty three thousand genes. But still no one knows, as yet, why a baby is born human and not a chimpanzee in spite of sharing ninety-eight percent of genes with chimps. It means that a variation of two percent explains the difference between a chimp and Miss Universe or the president of the United States. It demonstrates that very small differences in DNA can produce profoundly different results.

We are born with a set of genes and our genetic makeup is expressed in a myriad of ways such as height and weight, skin and eye color. It used to be thought that the information genes carried was fixed and unchangeable. Now we are finding that genes have switches that can be turned on or off, e.g. diabetes runs in families but there are a host of factors that turn it on.

The expression of a gene can be modified by the external environment and the internal milieu through habits, intentions and emotions. To a large extent, who we are, how we behave and our individual differences are a result of our genetic makeup. Genetics play a large role in when and how learning, growing, and development occurs. For example, children cannot walk before an age that is predetermined by their genome. However, while the genetic makeup of a child determines the age range for walking, environmental influences determine how early or late within that range the event will actually occur. In other words we can rephrase genes.

This process of rephrasing, changes the assembly and the structure of the "bits" of protein sequences.

Our genetic material influences who we become as people. We started with some basic characteristics and not a blank slate as Aristotle believed. Right from birth infants are unique individuals with a unique temperament. There are innate differences in readiness to smile, cry or vocalize, and energy levels. This temperament or trait is the raw material or foundation for personality. Observations of identical twins show that heredity has a significant effect on personality but not completely. Our genes weave a complex pattern working in concert with environmental and internal factors to express a personality trait.

The earliest concept of temperaments or humors probably originated in Mesopotamia, the cradle of ancient civilization. The notion of temperament was part of the theory of the four humors, with their corresponding four temperaments. This idea was expanded by Hippocrates and later Galen, correlating four fundamental body fluids or humors (blood, yellow bile, black bile, and phlegm) to four fundamental personality types (sanguine, choleric, melancholic and phlegmatic). An ideal temperament required a balance of the four healthy body fluids. Illness was thought to be caused by an imbalance in these four humors.

In the Nei Ching, which is an ancient Chinese medical text, there were five rather than four humors. Each humor has its seat in an organ e.g. happiness dwelt in the heart, sorrow in the lungs and anger in the liver. Seasons of the year, periods of life, geographic regions and occupations also influenced the nature of the humors formed. This viewpoint gave a more holistic understanding of life compared to Western medicine with its reductionist views, that every complex phenomenon can be completely understood and reduced to a simple component.

Temperament is that pattern of characteristic thoughts, feelings, and behaviors that distinguishes one person from another and that persists over time and situations. It arises from within the individual and remains fairly consistent throughout life. In psychology, temperament refers to those aspects of an individual's personality, which are often regarded as innate rather than learned. David Wechsler defines it as a global capacity to act purposefully, to think rationally, and to deal effectively with the environment. Temperament diminishes in importance as the personality becomes more developed.

We see differences in temperament in infants and young children that are present at birth or at least very early on in child development. We see differences in emotion, activity and attention. This childhood temperament continues into adulthood, influencing behavior and adjustment throughout life. Essentially, people act in the same ways or similar ways in a variety of situations.

However, we can transform our own temperaments with awareness and intelligent choices to shape our personalities. Having a role model helps in determining the characteristics we aspire to. Recognizing one's own personality, with tools such as Myers-Briggs personality types gives us a template that we can work from to realize our aspirations.

Intelligence is a complex trait influenced by many genetic and environmental factors. Studies show that—twenty to forty percent of childhood IQ (Intelligence Quotient) is due to genetic factors. However, we know little about the specific genes responsible for mental abilities or the factors responsible for expression of these genes. Identical twins growing up in the same family have highly correlated IQ scores. Adopted children who were moved to a better environment show striking increases in IQ. Nevertheless, heredity may limit the maximum IQ attained in spite of ideal conditions.

Intellect is a term that refers to the ability of the mind to solve problems, to think in a logical way and understand things quickly. Intellect appraises how we form meaningful patterns, and predicts educational ability with socially important outcomes. Howard Gardner in his book "Frames of Mind" outlines eight forms of intelligences ranging from verbal to musical, mathematical and people skills. With this range and complexity of the human intellect, every person has an intellect in one or more of these domains and no one should ever feel stupid!!

In the early nineteenth century, Samuel G Morton claimed that he could predict the intellectual ability of a race by measuring skull size. Morton erroneously believed that the skull size of a race determined their intellectual ability. A large skull meant a large brain and high intellectual capacity. He used his biased skull measurements as evidence to argue in favor of a racial hierarchy which put Caucasians on the top rung and Africans on the bottom. His theory, unfortunately, was exploited by those who favored slavery in the United States. It took many conscience-driven activists to right this wrong. It was their inner sense of what was right (or wrong) that impelled them toward right action.

This inner feeling or voice acting as a guide to the rightness or wrongness of one's behavior, is the voice of conscience. Conscience is equivalent to the superego in Freud's theory. When standards of the conscience are not followed we get punished internally by guilt feelings. Conscience functions as an internal parent. Although the capacity for conscience is probably genetically determined, it is developed by the reward/punishment behaviors of parents and later by society and culture. These factors are internalized, becoming individualized with both conscious and unconscious elements involving complex neural processing. At the highest level, conscience is refined by universal concepts of justice, equality and respect for the individual.

In Walt Disney's *Pinocchio* (a children's morality tale), Pinocchio's nose grows longer and longer when he fails to heed his conscience, caricatured as Jiminy Cricket. The character of Atticus, in Harper Lee's *To Kill a Mocking Bird*, says that he has to live with himself before he can live with others; and that a person's conscience does not abide by majority rule.

Buddha links the positive aspect of *conscience* to a pure heart and a calm, well-directed mind: *"when the mind is face to face with the Truth, a self-luminous spark of thought is revealed at the inner core of ourselves and, by analogy, all reality."* Dietrich Bonhoeffer, during his imprisonment by the Nazis in World War II, stated that conscience came from a depth beyond will and reason.

The Roman Emperor Marcus Aurelius wrote in his *Meditations* that "*conscience was the human capacity to live by rational principles that were congruent with the true, tranquil and harmonious nature of our mind and thereby that of the Universe.*"

A good conscience is associated with feelings of integrity, psychological wholeness and peacefulness. It is said that no pillow is softer than a clear conscience.

Charles Darwin considered that *conscience* evolved in humans to resolve conflicts between competing natural impulses relating to self-preservation or safety of a family or community. This inner conflict is often depicted as an angel representing conscience, and the devil representing temptation.

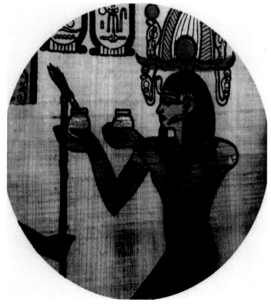

In Greek mythology, Eudemon was regarded as the good spirit or angel, and the evil Cacodemon was its opposing spirit.

In Islamic literature, there are two personal companions with each individual; one from the angels and another from the Jinn (spirits). The angel drives the individual to do good and obey God while that from the Jinn does the opposite. In Freudian terms, the Angel represents the super-ego (the source of self-censorship), counterbalanced by the Devil representing the id (the primal, instinctive desires of the individual).

Most religions see conscience as a judgment of reason or an internal "voice of God" that encourages a person to do the right thing and to avoid wrongdoing. On occasion our conscience behooves us to take a stand on positions that may be unpopular or even dangerous.

Catholics are exhorted to examine their conscience daily and seek absolution at confession. A sincere conscience presumes one is attentively seeking the truth from authentic sources. Nevertheless, Thomas Hobbes cautions that even opinions formed in good conscience can be potentially erroneous and not necessarily indicates absolute knowledge or truth.

Aquinas claimed *"it was weak will that allowed a non-virtuous man to choose a principle allowing pleasure ahead of one requiring moral constraint."* One with a weak or poorly developed conscience is incapable of balancing their own needs with those of others. A weak conscience leads to criminal or antisocial behavior whereas an overly harsh conscience results in unbearable guilt and rigidity.

Medical Applications

The belief that we are born with fixed genes no longer holds true. It is now recognized that the environment can induce mutations and alter genes. These mutations can arise from the internal environment just as much as the external.

Genetic testing has allowed the diagnosis of many diseases such as cystic fibrosis and neurofibromatosis. Down's syndrome can be detected as early as ten weeks in a pregnancy. Genetic engineering, by identifying and splicing or silencing genes is an exciting, though controversial, arena of research for potential cures for some genetic disorders.

The University of Iowa research center is working on a "bio patch" that inserts genetic instructions directly into cells to repair damaged bone. This exciting new technology can potentially be used to heal virtually any damaged tissue.

At each end of the chromosomes are stretches of DNA called telomeres that act as protective caps, much like the caps on live copper wires. They shield the ends of our chromosomes from fraying and sticking to each other. Each time our cells divide and the DNA is copied, these telomeres wear down and get shorter. When they get too short, structural integrity weakens, the cells age and die quicker. A body's enzyme called telomerase protects and rebuilds /elongates the telomeres to some degree. Oxidative stress, cortisol and inflammation break down the telomeres faster. Feeling stressed (even perceived stress) damages our health and ages us.

In recent years, shorter telomeres have become associated with a broad range of age related diseases, including many forms of cancer, stroke, vascular dementia, cardiovascular disease, obesity, osteoporosis and diabetes. Life style changes such as diet, exercise, stress management and social support may result in longer telomeres. Apparently meditation, by increasing levels of telomerase, repairs telomeres and slows down the aging process.

Meditative Exercise

Take a walk on a sandy beach or a boardwalk. Smell the salty air and hear the plaintive cry of the seagulls. Watch the birds in the air glide, soar and swoop, doing what they do without a care, or concern. They serve an essential purpose on this planet, scavenging and disposing of organic litter that pose a health threat to humans.

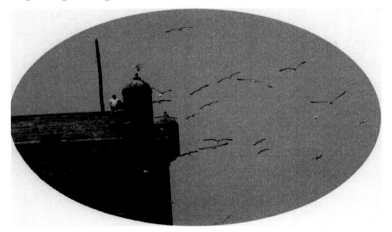

Essaouira, Morrocco

Although humans are genetically programmed in many ways to function and survive on this planet there is a vast untapped potential for growth and change superior to the animal kingdom.

How often have you considered the genetic makeup of your predecessors and woefully expressed the same fate awaiting you. How has that colored your life? Look beyond this belief and own that it does not have to be so, that you are the creator of your own health, and that even genetic change is possible. Experience the freedom that comes from absorbing and assimilating this thought.

Identify your own temperament utilizing any of the personality questionnaires available on the world wild web. The broad range of temperaments and personalities provide richness to society. Recognize the differences in others around you. Accept them at their level of intellect and function for who they are. Let each grow at their own pace. Everyone has their place, as much as our winged sanitation engineers, the seagulls, in the nature of things.

Chapter 25
OUR HISTORY

"Whoever wishes to foresee the future must consult the past; for human events ever resemble those of preceding times. This arises from the fact that they are produced by men who ever have been, and ever shall be, animated by the same passions, and thus they necessarily have the same results."

—Machiavelli

Our history colors our perspective, and the way we express ourselves through our behavior. Our experiences, starting from the time in the womb, configure our brains. Warm, welcoming, accepting messages set the stage for a secure, well balanced child. This influence continues during infancy and throughout life as an ongoing process. The people and events of our past shape us into who we are.

The culture we grew up in and what happens to us stays in our memory and forms our ego and shapes our beliefs. The brain is not simply a receiving station for sensory signals. Our emotions, memories, moods, and beliefs constantly influence what we see, hear, and feel and how we respond to our biosphere. Our sense of the world is a creation of the brain and the mind. Similar events may be experienced quite differently, from day to day and at different times of our life. The limbic processes receive the messages from sight, touch and sounds, and form our expectations of the nature of our world.

Customs, manners and social life are expressed by people as a representation of their culture. Culture is a traditional way to pass on societal practices from one generation to the next and these patterns of behavior are generally observed by the group. For example, in Chinese culture of filial piety, children are expected to look after their parents in their old age. The unconscious bonds of our own culture, inevitably impact our perceptions of and reactions to the world.

In our multicultural world, we have to make sense of another person's beliefs and behaviors in the context of their culture. Anne Fadiman in *The Spirit Catches You and You Fall Down*, tells the story of a Hmong child, Lia, who was afflicted with seizures as an infant. The Hmong consider seizures as evidence of a higher power that allows epileptics to see things beyond normal beings. Epileptics often become shamans in their culture. This cultural belief resulted in the resistance of the parents to adequately treat the child with anti-seizure medications. Failure, on the part of the caregivers, to understand the culture led to mismanagement of Lia's care. Even well-educated people, can strongly cling to their beliefs, and act on these beliefs even when it is detrimental to self or others.

Holding on to beliefs, narrows one's experience and expression for life.

Beliefs can be changed either through a life-changing experience or a thoughtful process of questioning and rejection/modification of held beliefs. As the Dalai Lama has said, the authority of scriptures cannot prevail over an understanding based on reason and experience. This nugget of wisdom forces us to rethink the authority of scriptures. In other words, the filter of belief and preconception that we look through is often faulty and not necessarily the truth.

> *"Believers filter the world to remain consistent with the non-negotiable principles of their faith"*
> —Roy Baumeister.

We focus only on the facts and viewpoints of what we already believe ignoring and silencing the cognitive dissonance. We experience reality by what we perceive. Only through the prism of objectivity and contemplation can we see things as they are, and then be able to express our convictions with greater confidence.

By living fully and welcoming all that nature and others around us can show us, we can change our beliefs leading to growth and greater personal satisfaction.

Beliefs should evolve as we gain new experiences and knowledge to allow for better choices and actions. Undoubtedly, there are fundamental similarities in the structure of human thought the world over. There is an almost universal belief in the existence of God or higher power of some kind as an attempt to explain the inexplicable, or the ultimate reality.

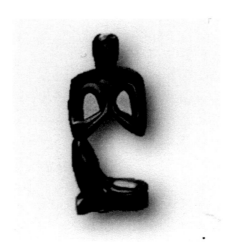

The concept of God is a product of human evolution as there is, deep in the human psyche, a need to explain and make sense of our existence and of the world we live in. For some it has been a presence that transformed their lives. Religions evolve to express that transforming guidance and to share beliefs and rituals.

Demasio, Newberg and others have done extensive research to determine if the religious impulse is rooted in the biology of the brain. To date, the research shows changes in the brain on MRI while meditating and during spiritual experiences. However, the reality of a god cannot be established by changes occurring in the brain.

Not surprisingly either, no difference is noted on MRI findings amongst subjects with different religious traditions. In other words, the general aspects of how we formulate our beliefs, and our spiritual experiences are relatively similar. The brain reconciles crucial existential problems through the same neural pathways irrespective of the belief system.

Although studies do not reflect on whether God exists or not, undeniably there is that *"unseen order"* in the universe that is beyond our comprehension. Belief in an unseen order has added awe and enchantment to life—from the appreciation of the delicate petals of a flower to the spectacular sunsets. After centuries of research and thought we still have incomplete answers as to how our own minds and bodies work.

The Emerald Tablet, an ancient Arabic work, believed to be written between the sixth and eighth centuries, gives us a sense of this underlying mystery: *"as all things are made from one…. the father of it is the sun, the mother the moon. The wind bore it in the womb. Its nurse is the earth, the mother of all perfection."*

Religious traditions offer teachings that allow people to express life and to live it more fully. Religious literature is full of complexities, filled with art, poetry, insight and inspiration. Religions foster attitudes and qualities that help people deal with difficulties and death, and influences the life one leads. Most mainstream religions capitalize on the fear of death and a promise of a life to come.

Beliefs have a deep impact on how we think, behave and act. Most individuals believe in the religion they were taught in childhood.

Religious beliefs, intertwined with secular beliefs, ultimately affects everything we do, and permeates every part of our lives. What we believe influences our thinking; what we think translates into our words and actions and eventually our habits. To break our destructive habits we have to source it back to our beliefs. Change our belief, change the way we behave.

The personal search for meaning and connection is one's spirituality. Authenticity is listening to one's innermost convictions in evaluating experiences instead of mindlessly following tradition, authority or the majority. Faith is an inner conviction that is experienced rather than belief in what another has said. It is not stagnant and can change as we evolve and grow in wisdom.

Those who remain unsure of their beliefs and desires generally feel insecure and confused about themselves and the future.

Charismatic leaders, politicians and the media can form or change beliefs through authority and repetition. Misguided interpretation leads to a fanatical *"one and only true way."* Consider the fifty million people killed in Russia to further the cause of communism or the untold waste of life in the Holocaust as a result of false belief.

The subconscious mind may contain beliefs, feelings or experiences that occurred in the past that are long forgotten and that we do not normally access. These underlying feelings and thoughts are stored in the form of memories, which often affect how we behave. Memories are not so much objective snapshots as they are subjective reconstructs influenced by our particular thoughts and feelings at the time we form the memory. Memory involves receiving and processing information followed by storage and subsequent retrieval on command. Comparable to placing information on a clipboard, short term memories are temporary and easily forgotten. Incoming information is sifted for relevance and content and then stored by creating a record of the encoded information as long term memory. The brain does a 'save' to the hard drive.

"Things that have it easy die early in nature. Plants and trees that have to fight through adversity, they have the longest life, their mettle tested and hardened by constant challenge. In nature, adversity breeds longevity."
—Michael Modzelewski

So too in our brains, strong, positive emotions connected with an experience is more likely to be stored and more easily accessed or retrieved.

Our brains seem to have no limits on storage of experiences; experiences that are cherished, forgotten, ignored or avoided. The complex reconstructions of our past are retrieved by recollection of the information subconsciously or at will. That memory is expressed at the conscious level. The scars of negative experiences remain balanced by the treasury of beautiful memories to be revisited time and time again. We cannot change the past but we have control of the hold it has on us.

Research has revealed that the hippocampus is vital for memory consolidation and retrieval. The hippocampus links the thinking brain (neocortical systems) with the feeling brain (limbic systems). In addition there is a network of brain regions involved in supporting memories of our personal experiences. It's a dynamic process where every factor influences the other so it is difficult to tease apart the components. Damage to the hippocampus has a devastating impact on the ability to form new memories and compromises our recollection of the past. Significant gaps in our knowledge remain, and we do not quite know how activity across millions of hippocampal neurons supports a person's lifetime of experiences. But we do know that excessive or prolonged stress (with prolonged cortisol) may hurt memory storage. Incidentally, unresolved painful events and memories are carried in our bodies, muscles, nervous system and respiratory system as fixed patterns which may explain the syndrome of fibromyalgia.

Just as memory involves a host of complex synaptic connections in the prefrontal cortex so too does the ego. We all know what ego is but it is a concept that is hard to wrap one's brain around. It is one of the most maligned words in our vocabulary. But in actuality, we need to have a healthy ego.

A baby does not have a sense of the ego when born. Infants gradually develop awareness of their bodies and the reality beyond their bodies. The ego is shaped by life's happenings. It is a self-construct of what has happened, what has been said to us and what the mind has perceived over time. Our ego identity is constantly changing and growing, due to new experiences and information acquired in our daily interactions with others. As we grow we form a mental image of who we are. This personal identity gives us an integrated and cohesive sense of self.

It is, however, an illusory sense of self, created by identification with the processes of the mind.

The ego is not our total self. Carl Jung describes it as an off-center circle contained within the whole. We base our ego identity on situations, circumstances, achievement's, memory, perception, learning and intelligence. It is our opinion of our own worth developed through social interaction. In turn, our ego exercises a strong influence on our perception and how we express ourselves in our world, and most of the time we are unaware of this influence. It comes from an unconscious need within that is concerned with our safety, reputation, personal interest, and survival. Every human being is a unique individual and there is a powerful drive to maintain this individuality. Because of this we tend to go to extremes to defend perceived threats to the ego.

Our version of reality is skewed by the ego's agenda to feel better about ourselves. The ego makes up for our deficiencies and insecurities by pretending to be more important or better than everyone else. The ego thrives on being the best and fosters a need to be right and to be in control. The ego is never satisfied and is always craving more. People with overinflated egos are blinded by feelings of superiority. The ego runs amok when it loses touch with true self or center.

A poorly developed ego leads to low self-esteem or psychological anorexia. An unhealthy ego keeps us detached from our surroundings and society. Understanding that our ego identity is illusory and not our true selves, helps us to step back to find meaningful connections. Psychiatrist R.D. Laing states, *"True sanity entails….. the dissolution of the normal ego…..The ego being the servant of the divine* (or true self), *no longer its betrayer."* Subjugating the ego to true self enhances our self-worth and makes for a richer, healthier and meaningful life.

As we journey through our lives, everything that happens, every person we talk to, affects the way we ultimately shape our behavior and express ourselves. Lessons from the past are relevant in decision-making in daily life, and strongly affects how we live our lives. But our identity is not defined by that history; we can, at any moment in time, change our destructive beliefs and behavior patterns and resolve to walk down more enlightened, brighter paths.

Medical Applications

Holding fast to cultural beliefs without due consideration can lead to harm as in the case of the Hmong child, Lia. Cultural expectations of weight and body image in Western society lead to anorexia nervosa. Cultural fears about sexual overindulgence have been the basis for Koro or an acute anxiety reaction seen in Southeast Asia.

Among the Cree Indians of North America, minor gastrointestinal symptoms can lead to anxiety, for fear of being transformed into a 'wihtigo'—a giant monster that eats human flesh.

By exploring the past, psychotherapy can bring to light issues that play a part in maladaptive behaviors. People with Borderline Personality Disorder characteristically lack a strong sense of identity. An over inflation of the ego leads to a Narcissistic Personality Disorder characterized by grandiose self-importance and extreme preoccupation with self. The capacity to see the other is lost, resulting in psychologic and interpersonal problems. Reality is replaced by fantasy, delusions and unrealistic megalomaniac beliefs.

Amnesia, a memory disorder, occurs as the result of brain injury and occasionally emotional trauma. Alzheimer's and other causes of dementia leads to progressive memory loss that disrupts daily life in families.

In mental illnesses such as Alzheimer's disease, schizophrenia and autism, there is a distortion of the personal self and a lack of insight. The sadness of these disease is captured in Oliver Sacks' book, *The Man Who Mistook His Wife for a Hat*. Patients with these mental states lack the insight to see their deficiencies. The distortion in thinking that occurs is incomprehensible to caretakers and contacts. The patient's incapacity as well as the care-givers difficulty in grasping what is going on in the afflicted mind makes for tough situations. It takes detachment and compassion to deal with the day to day challenges posed in caring for the mentally ill.

Meditative Exercise
Spend time with and get to know someone who comes from a different culture. Explore the similarities and differences in belief

systems. Let go of preconceived prejudices and judgments. Find value and uniqueness in the other. Without judgement make a conscious effort to appreciate another's inner world of thoughts, feelings and intentions.

Find a place to be quiet and comfortable. Light a candle and play soft soothing music. Create an atmosphere of peace and tranquility.

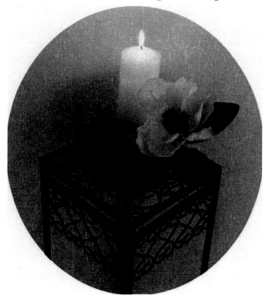

Gently regulate your breathing, inhaling and exhaling equally, pausing between the inhalation and exhalation. Drift into the center of your being. Allow yourself to examine and question the concepts and beliefs that have caused pain, guilt or hurt. You have the freedom to let go of repetitive, self-defeating messages. Feel the release in your throat and around your heart as you make this choice. As you release the negativity, you create more space for positive, loving and caring energy.

Allow yourself to enjoy wonderful, precious memories of your past. Enjoy the sense of pleasure as you relive these moments. As you review the past, see your life as a continuum of lessons learned, challenges met and endeavors fulfilled. Every life is a journey of discovery.

Chapter 26
THE EXTRINSICS

"Words are a pretext. It is the inner bond that draws one person to another, not words."

—Jalaluddin Rumi

"Real knowledge is to know the extent of one's ignorance."

—Confucius

Before language, one "read" the other through nonverbal body signals, gestures, facial expressions and grunts. As civilization progressed, grunts transitioned to words and subsequently the written word; the art of language flowered. Language is what defines humans.

Everyone on earth initially spoke the same language. But when they started building a tower to reach the sky, God intervened and scrambled their speech. As a result they could not understand each other, and they were scattered over the face of the earth; or so it says in the book of Genesis in the Christian Bible.

Language has become a complex means of expression to encompass ideas and abstract concepts. Wikipedia defines language as a system of communication that enables humans to exchange verbal or symbolic utterances. This definition stresses the social functions of language. Humans use language to express themselves and the mind creates meaning association. Two areas in the brain are crucially implicated in language processing. Comprehension and understanding of language take place in the upper back convolution of the temporal lobe in the dominant cerebral hemisphere known as Wernicke's area.

Expression of language is processed by Broca's area, located in the back and lower part of the frontal lobe in the dominant hemisphere. The non-dominant hemisphere seems to appreciate the abstract in language such as tonality and cadence.

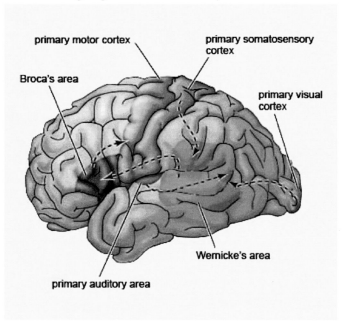

Image taken from The Brain from Top to Bottom under copyleft

Language is the way the brain attempts to symbolically and coherently express and explain its abstract thoughts and ideas to itself and to the outside world. The critical period for language is up to seven years of age. Children learn language by imitation from their elders and peers and pass that knowledge to their own children. Thus language is dependent on the community in which one grows up. Society does not function without language. Oral language is vital to the process of socialization.

Humans have the ability to learn any language, and it is not uncommon for people to be fluent in multiple languages. In this day and age we need global ways of communication. With technology, the internet, and auto-translate functions, we are reaching this objective.

The power of language can be used to communicate, instruct, influence, inspire and entertain. True maturity of expression is marked by thoughtfulness, consideration and honesty. As the saying goes, *"Say what you mean and mean what you say."* Articulation asserts one's needs and is an expression of who we are as unique individuals. Our ability to express ideas, hopes, disappointments and desires, contributes to living an effective life.

We all have experienced the power of words. Innocent little things one says can set off a chain reaction that becomes explosive. Well-chosen words can speak to the soul or move us to tears. Words are seeds that land in hearts and minds. We can choose to cultivate positive expressions and responses. A skillful use of words, whether spoken or written, goes a long way in building relationships.

The need for a permanent record of information and thoughts led to the invention of writing. Writing adds permanence to our words much as a sculpture does to an artist's creative vision. Writing, as we know it today, was a gradual process starting out as symbols or pictographs. Chinese script or Egyptian hieroglyphics etched in stone, leather or papyrus could be stored, passed on or retrieved at a future date. This early writing gradually evolved to alphabets—equating sounds to symbols. Writing helps organize our thoughts, giving focus and direction. Hence the use of journaling as a psychotherapeutic tool.

With the advent of print, large bodies of knowledge could be stored for posterity and shared. Thanks to the internet, access to this body of knowledge is readily available with just a mouse-click.

Knowledge is stored in the neocortex. We use what we have learned as building blocks to acquire and expand our knowledge about something new. With the vast pool of available knowledge, it is impossible to know all there is to know. Besides, all knowledge is incomplete at best. Knowledge can be taught, read or experienced. A wise man once said *that not every reader becomes a leader, but every leader is a reader.* Possession of facts, ideas, truths, information and data opens the door to a universe of truth and wisdom. The silos of data and information are different for each individual depending on their interests. What we learn shapes our lives and the kind of person we become. Life is a process of learning and growing in understanding.

> *"It ain't what you don't know that gets you in trouble;*
> *it's what you know for sure that ain't so"*
> —Mark Twain

An artist or musician spends years learning the basic principles. It is only with practice they become skilled at what they do. Mastery of language is no different. Mastery comes from structured, focused study. The learning process can be an enjoyable never-ending journey. We can explore areas of knowledge we lack. We can explore the world of the written word with an open mind to find fascination in mundane things.

Practice improves our skill. From the age of six to eleven, children develop a sense of competence and belief in their skills. Encouragement from parents, teachers, or peers play an important role in this growth. Associating with people who challenge us stretches our thinking.

Plato and Aristotle and the mediaeval universities held that grammar, rhetoric, and logic were the skills that had to be acquired for effective writing, reading, speaking, and listening.

The brain adapts to a new skill according to your intent and desire. Skill is defined as "the ability to use one's knowledge effectively and readily." Skills can be purely technical like mechanics and surgery; cognitive like analytical reasoning and planning; or aptitudes utilizing emotional intelligence to manage relationships, forge networks, and build rapport.

Whatever our skills, it is important to be realistic and learn to know our assets and liabilities; strengths and weaknesses. We need to have a belief in our own abilities to handle the tasks set before us. We have to accept ourselves with all our gifts as well as our faults. Having a firm grasp of our capabilities we are less likely to set ourselves up to fail. A person who lacks self-awareness is apt to make decisions that bring on inner turmoil by overreaching or compromising values.

"Your work is to discover your work and then with all your heart to give yourself to it."
—Buddha

We spend a considerable part of our lives in the world of work. We should focus time, energy, training and research on pursuits that complement our natural abilities, interests and passions. Line your ducks in a row and get the geese to fly in formation. Incorporating language, knowledge and skill in projects that have meaning consistent with our core values, we find our vocation. Rumi poetically says *"Let yourself be silently drawn by the stronger pull of what you really love."* David Spangler describes it as finding a resonance in one's life that allows the full expression and connection with the larger whole.

Our career path is never set in stone. We have the ability to forge and reinvent ourselves at any stage. Our brains are adaptable and allow us choices to influence events in our life; this is the adventure of becoming uniquely ourselves.

Experiencing resonance, meaning and fulfillment in our chosen field is a definite bonus. Positive experiences originate from the way tasks are approached and performed rather than the task itself. The nervous system is conditioned to move to pleasant and away from unpleasant at the limbic level of functioning. With the frontal cortex we can reframe the jobs we dislike and change the feeling to enjoyment by giving it a fresh perspective. We are at liberty to choose our response and free ourselves from the tyranny of the amygdala.

The Tao Te Ching states, *"See simplicity in the complicated. Achieve greatness in little things."* The mundane in daily living is transformed by attitude, depth of engagement and dedication. The Japanese Tea ceremony is a simple art of making tea but when done as a ritual, it is infused with sacredness and meaning. This awareness is also brought out in Thoreau's *Walden* where the most ordinary actions are made sacred. The work we do should not be considered simply as a "job" , but one's contribution to the community and, by extension, keeping the world at peace and harmony. An employee works in a factory cranking out nuts and bolts day after day. When we realize the integrity of an airplane and the safety of the passengers on board depends on this repetitive task done well, the importance of this work cannot be stressed enough. Our primary mission is to enjoy the earth and its beauty and not get caught up in unnecessary gloom and despair. Dance at work and be filled with life.

The Buddhist way is to do the work well with diligence, without attachment or push to make it meaningful. Being active in home and community fosters feelings of contribution and involvement in the world and with others.

Our vocation allows the time and resources for what we need and want. Money is the current artificial tool for barter. Being overly attached to these wrinkled pieces of exchange gives us angst. Be astute in the use of money that we slog our whole lives for, but keep it in perspective and use money for the enrichment of life. *Slide down rainbows and slosh in mud puddles.*

Language, knowledge, skills and vocation; these are the accoutrements by which we express a part of us. These acquired, extrinsic factors, although essential for existence and survival in our society, are not the essence of our identities. They are appendages that can easily detract us from the essential nature of self.

Medical Applications

When a stroke injures the frontal regions of the left hemisphere, different kinds of language problems can occur depending on the extent of the damage. Injury to Broca's area leads to expressive aphasia, a state where people know what they want to say, but cannot verbalize it. They are able to understand what is being said to them, but cannot communicate it to others.

Damage to Wernicke's area leads to difficulty processing what is coming in, or receptive aphasia, where the person can hear speech or read writing, but cannot understand the meaning of the message. It is like they are listening to a foreign language. Their own speech may be disturbed, stringing together a series of meaningless words or made up words. With therapy, communication can be improved using gestures, drawing or even special software on computers.

It is important to have a realistic view of one's abilities. A mismatch in one's abilities and job requirements can lead to misery, anxiety and depression.

Before striving to make a living is done with, it is important to plan for retirement and have something to do with newfound time. Identifying too much with their roles at work, many retirees suffer from depression and go to pieces as a result of their new circumstance.

Approach retirement as a period of discovery and time to enjoy family and the beauty around you and experience life anew.

"In the end it is not the years in your life that counts; it's the life in your years."

—Abe Lincoln

Meditative Exercise

Settle in your quiet spot. It could be a favorite couch in your living room. Or it could be a quiet area under a shady tree, or by the water's edge.

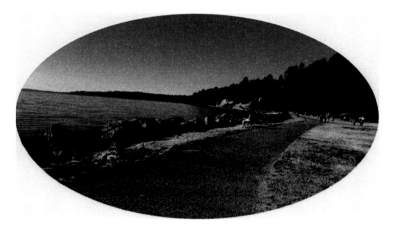

Des Moines, WA

Bring awareness of your surroundings to your mind. The gentle breeze rustling through the leaves, the waves lapping on the rocks, or the soft fabric of the comfy couch. Let the awareness then rest on your breath; appreciate the nuances of each inhalation and each exhalation. Let your next in-breath circle up your spine to the top of your head and then, in the out-breath, wash down the front of your chest completing a *"heavenly circle,"* a circle of safety and protection.

Now bring to mind an interaction with someone who speaks a different language. Examine the attitude with which this person was approached. Was there a tendency to dismiss or belittle this person without exploring or considering the skills and knowledge he or she has? Switch gears and recreate the encounter, with openness to the skills he or she has to offer. Connect at the level of soul, beyond words and language. Watch the play of the mind and conversation with self as you journal these thoughts.

Apply this insight and change of perspective at work and in daily interactions.

Chapter 27
OUR POTENTIAL

"If you think you are too small to have an impact, Try going to bed with a mosquito."

—African proverb

"Without leaps of imagination or dreaming, we lose the excitement of possibilities."

—Gloria Steinem

Imagination is the process of forming new images in the mind not perceived by the senses, but may be influenced by past experience. Imagined images are seen with the "mind's eye."

In ancient times inspiration and creativity was thought to be metaphysical and "sent from God(s)." We can appreciate why scriptural texts are replete with "the voice of God." According to Greek mythology, the Nine Muses were nine goddesses—the daughters of Zeus and Mnemosyne— that gave artists, philosophers, and individuals the necessary inspiration for creation. We still say we are "channeling the muse" when searching for creative inspiration.

It was only after the age of enlightenment, in the sixteenth century that the imagination was no longer relegated to the caprice of the gods. Isaac Newton's discovery that every motion on the ground or in space behaves in the same simple manner according to universally applicable, mathematical laws encouraged the concept of nature as an orderly domain. The concept that humankind can understand the laws of nature through the exercise of our own faculties opened the doors to innovation and modern science.

Child-development experts are recognizing the importance of imagination and the role it plays. Children with imagination are more creative, have greater social skills and understanding of the perspective of others. Opportunities to develop imagination is often found in play with paints, glue and crayons. Pretend play with costumes or being outdoors, exploring the woods or seeing a bird gliding through the sky, is fertile ground for the imagination. Imagination is the source of ideas and the beginning of creation. To quote Michelangelo, *"I saw the angel in the marble and carved until I set him free."* It was Thoreau's imagination that fired the creative life he led.

Imagination brings alive history and tales of other lands. As Albert Einstein says imagination takes one everywhere as opposed to logic that takes one from A to Z.

As adults we stagnate without imagination. A vivid inner realm of imagination, pushes us out of our habitual way of thinking. By simply watching television or reading fiction we become passive participants in someone else's stories. Solitude, with time and space to dream and reignite the inner child within, is essential to the imagination. Creativity is imagination put into action, forming something new.

Creativity can be analogous to pottery making which requires conscious attention to every step in the process. The word for "potter" in the Old Testament, *yatsar*, means "the one who forms." In the book of Genesis, God is pictured as forming man from the earth just as a potter forms his pots from clay. Clay must be prepared by kneading, thrown and shaped on a wheel; then fired in a kiln before cooling and glazing. Multiple variables, including temperature changes, ultimately define the finished product. There is a tension between control and letting go.

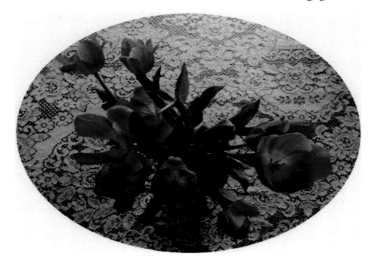

Ikebana is a creative Japanese art of flower arrangement showcasing nature and humanity. Stems, leaves and flowers, and attention to the spaces in between, form elegant contours that emphasize and enhance its natural beauty. It is a true expression of creativity to see common objects in a new way. Renowned photo journalist for National Geographic Dewitt Jones looks at the ordinary and sees the extraordinary. The result is his amazing, spectacular photography.

At the heart of every being is the capacity to be creative; whether it is an idea, a piece of music or finding hidden relationships to solve an everyday problem. We can find opportunities in the workplace, kitchen or backyards. We're all creative in our own little ways. It involves a variety of self-directed thought processes which can be learned. When we are creative we use more of our brains integrating our complex neuronal networks. Creativity happens when we align with our natural gifts, excite our natural curiosities and engage in play. The creative energy of the universe works through us.

Using MRI techniques, it has been found that a relaxed state of mind induced alpha waves in the brain correlating with greater insight and the creative potential. The creative process is an exercise of surrender; letting go and allowing ideas to percolate and transform into perfection. The brain is an ocean of endless connections, flexible and fluid, able to blend together concepts filed away in the dark recesses of the mind. Forming new connections leads to those lightning flashes of inspiration. Creativity can also be a time consuming and labor intensive process. A new idea is often not the end of the creative process. Milton Glaser's simple I love NY logo, has continued on: on cups, T-shirts, used and adapted in many innovative ways.

Our creative forces can stay stifled because of fear, especially fear of failure. Viewing failure as a learning experience we can build on it to further our goals.

Imagination and creativity accounts for the unprecedented breakthroughs in science and technology; from the first sharpened stick, to the wheel, to the space shuttle and to the micro-processor. Without imagination and creativity there would be no progress. We would be caught in the same groove.

Nietzsche writes of the ideal creative, independent, spiritual genius which he calls the *Übermensch or overman*. An overman's work of art is his own life, lived according to his own creative will. Will or volition is the conscious generation of intentions by which an individual decides on and commits to a particular course of action. It is defined as purposeful striving and is one of the primary human psychological functions.

Will, or volition, involves intention and a firm or unwavering determination to adhere to one's purpose. Intention is the deliberate desire to bring about a specific outcome.

One of the innate characteristics of children is their strength of will or willfulness which varies from child to child. It is part of their emotional and intellectual package built into their nature. They bring with them an individuality that is uniquely their own. Strong-willed kids are spirited and courageous with passionate feelings. They want to learn things for themselves rather than accept what others say, so they test limits over and over. Strong willed children can be a challenge when they're young, but they become terrific teens and young adults, given the right direction. Strong-willed kids often turn into adults with integrity, not easily swayed from their own viewpoints. Self-motivated and inner-directed, they go after what they want. These are the kids that through self-expression often become leaders to make a difference in the world someday.

A person's will is one of the most distinct parts of their mind, along with reason and understanding. It is said that genius is two percent inspiration and ninety-eight perspiration. With our will, we can reach beyond our boundaries and achieve heights not known before. Will or intent is especially important for people to act deliberately and make ethical decisions.

According to Buddhist teachings, Right Intention is part of the path to wisdom and the second aspect of the Eightfold Path. Doing the right thing with the right intent generally leads to success. The more we express and believe in our intentions and act on it, the more real they become. With intention we have a clear focus directing our thoughts and subconscious mind. Wayne Dyer, in his book *The Power of Intention*, talks about intention as a field of energy in the universe that we can access to allow the act of creation to take place. By focusing on our intention, we creatively strategize its realization. Dr. Emoto validates the power of positive thinking by demonstrating that human thoughts and intentions can alter physical reality, through his thought experiments on the geometric structure of water crystals.

Marcus Aurelius and other prominent thinkers have had lengthy dissertations regarding the role of free will vs. determinism or the doctrine that all events, including human action, transpire according to the universe's own plan.

Using functional MRI, neurologists correlate human action to brain function. With these techniques, the brain showed activity ten seconds before we become aware of our intentions and actions. In other words humans may not have full access to various internal neural processes. A subconscious factor initiates the process before we are aware of it. That unseen force is you, the thinker behind the thought, and the perceiver behind the perceived, and the doer behind the deed that champions freedom of will against a doctrine of predetermination.

Philosopher Walter Jackson Freeman III states that it is our intentional actions streaming into the world that changes it. He also states that it is the power of unconscious systems (or self) that is the agency in charge, not our awareness. It is through the intent of activists to change policies regarding women's rights, slavery and civil rights,(to name but a few) that has had the greatest impact on societal health; far greater than medications.

We can choose to be the "overman" living with a will or a life-affirming drive to express our full potential. We can think for ourselves or follow the herd instinct to be led by circumstances.

Choice is the mental faculty of conscious rational thinking by which one deliberately chooses or decides upon a course of action when options are available. Choice involves the use of reason to explore all options. We do not have to have it all figured out to move forward. There is some evidence that while multiple options have the potential to improve a person's welfare, sometimes too much choice confounds the mind and we shut down.

Depending too much on rational brain often leads to "over-thinking" and sometimes making the wrong decision. But wrong decisions can be corrected to effect a different outcome if we choose. We make choices on a daily basis—little ones or life changing ones. The moment of choice is a crossroad—to choose the path less travelled or the deeply furrowed trails. We often make choices based on our emotions. Better choices occur when reason, emotion and intuition are factored in.

In ancient Rome, men invoke Janus, as the god to point the way. He is usually depicted as having two faces, since he looks to the future from the past. He symbolizes the process of change from past to future, from one condition to another, from one vision to another.

Besides using oracles and shamans and their tools to help in making decisions in personal lives, choices were made using signs in nature—the wind pattern, the star in the sky, the movement of birds. Amongst the Hindus in India, astrology played a large part in determining marriage compatibility and auspicious dates. Using three coins tossed six times and based on sixty-four hexagrams, the I Ching system of divination is still consulted to give answers to questions posed. Imaginative and creative interpretations from the imagery on tarot cards determines significance and pathways to move through a situation.

Ultimately, when we are aligned with our essence and trust the flow of the universe we will proceed on the right path. We are the only ones who have the total perception of ourselves to make our choices to either hold back or move forward. In the long run we are shaped by the choices we make.

During a boat trip up the Isis with a few colleagues and their three young daughters, Charles L. Dodgson tells the girls a story about a bored little girl named Alice who goes looking for an adventure and falls down a rabbit hole. Dodgson's imagination and creativity took the girls into a fantasy world with strange but lovable characters. The girls loved it and asked Dodgson to write it down. Dodgson chose to comply, perfected the tale and with will and determination brought to fruition the timeless classic *"Alice in Wonderland"* under the pseudonym of Lewis Carroll.

"The Possible's slow fuse…lit by the Imagination."
—Emily Dickinson.

We can imagine the life we want and use our creativity to achieve it with will and choice. Each present moment is a crossroad in time; the time to forge our destiny. Now is the time to realize our potential on the anvil of the past with both the intrinsic and extrinsic tools. Deeds done, loves lost, sufferings survived with dignity and courage are full silos for actualising possibilities and fulfilling dreams. And yes, we can laugh when we fall off the stepping stones into the river but delight in the times that we made it across.

Medical Applications

There is a link between creative expression and healing or coping with life's health related challenges. A sense of mastery and achievement using creative expression boosts the immune system and enhances well-being.

Creativity hastens recovery from infections and injuries, and reduces pain from chronic conditions. Poetry, writing, art, or music therapy taps into one's own experience to transform and heal. These art forms are being used therapeutically among cancer survivors with remarkable results.

Meditative Exercise

Meditation frees the mind from old circuits allowing fresh new ideas to blossom. Find your favorite place to be. Quieten the mind, focusing on your breath. Feel the silence and the opening of your heart and mind. Explore ways to express creative living whether with family or at work.

Choose an art form that speaks to you to explore and understand what is inside of you and to grow as a person. Play the music that is in you.

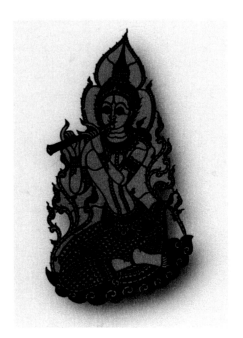

Let your imagination run wild. Harness the universal creative energy and create freely. Pay attention to day dreams and fantasies to harness new ideas and insights. The end result is of no import, only the process.

With imagination and creativity paint your life as an exquisite, unique work of art.

CHAKRA 6

THE THIRD EYE CHAKRA
TWO PETALS (CLUSTERS) OF CONSCIOUSNESS

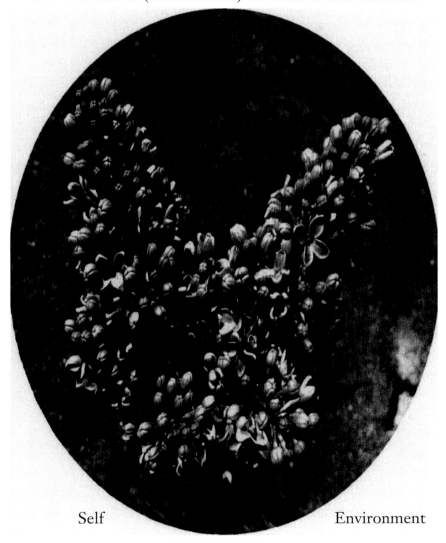

Self   Environment

Chapter 28
TWO PETALS OF CONSCIOUSNESS

"A new consciousness is developing which sees the earth as a single organism and recognizes that an organism at war with itself is doomed."

—Carl Sagan

Cosmos: A Personal Voyage

"Nothing gives life more purpose than the realization that every moment in consciousness is a precious and fragile gift."

—Steven Pinker.

The color associated with the sixth chakra is violet which has the highest vibration in the visible spectrum of light. It is a secondary color connecting red and blue on a color chart. The related colors are indigo and purple. These form the VIP colors (Violet Indigo and Purple). These are the colors of royalty and nobility. It combines the energy and strength of red with the spirituality and integrity of blue. Violet is the symbol of spiritual attainment, self-mastery, and wisdom. The violet gemstone *Amethyst* is often set in the episcopal bishop's ring and worn as amulets by medieval European soldiers as protection in battle.

This third eye chakra is associated with the pineal gland which resembles a tiny pine cone located near the center of the brain, between the two cerebral hemispheres. The cells of the pineal gland have a strong resemblance to the photoreceptor cells of the eye. Some evolutionary biologists believe that the vertebrate pineal cells possess a common evolutionary pathway with retinal cells, hence the "third eye."

"Close both eyes to see with the other eye"
—Rumi

Many cultures conceptualize the third eye as a mystical inner eye that can access intuition, clarity and insight. It is said to expand our awareness and inspire high ideals; connecting us to a higher consciousness, leading to a transformation of the soul. It symbolizes a state of enlightenment. It is not determined if these states are related to dimethyltryptamine, a hallucinogenic substance, thought to be secreted by the pineal gland.

Taoism teaches that the third eye, also called the mind's eye, is one of the main meridian of energy centers of the body separating the left and right hemispheres of the body. The third eye symbol is used in many ancient Asian meditation practices such as yoga, qigong and Aikido. Yoga promotes meditative practices to achieve a state of consciousness free from thought, with awareness of its own nature. A bright dot of red color, known as a bindi, applied in the center of the forehead between the eyebrows is worn in South Asia representing the third eye. Focusing on this spot is believed to strengthen concentration, awakening into the infinite mystery and beauty of life.

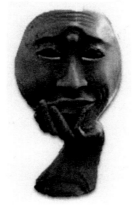

Egyptian myth has it that the eye of goddess Isis radiates a direct energetic connection to the Ultimate Creator. This "all-seeing eye" , often surrounded by light rays enclosed by a triangle, represents the eye of God watching over mankind. This symbol has been adopted as the Great Seal of the United States and is seen on the back of the American dollar bill. The unfinished pyramid with thirteen steps, represents the original thirteen states and the future growth of the country.

In many religious traditions, the concept of the third eye is a metaphor for non-dualistic mystical thinking. Father Richard Rohr refers to this level of awareness as "having the mind of Christ."

This association of the third eye with mystical awakening or enlightenment, and higher states of consciousness is the essence of the sixth chakra. According to Eckhart Tolle, we can be conscious without thinking but cannot think without consciousness.

Some have suggested the existence of a cosmic consciousness, asserting that consciousness is actually the "ground of all being" or an invisible intelligence that weaves the fabric of life. It is speculated that consciousness is the primary creative force in the cosmos, all things being ultimately derived from a Universal power or deity. Consciousness is often described as light coming from this eternal source. In Mahayana Buddhism the Universal mind or consciousness has no beginning and no end.

Astronaut Edgar Mitchell said of his experience in space that he felt an *"overwhelming sense of universal connectedness. I perceived the universe as in some way conscious."*

In medical terminology there are five states of consciousness—sleep, dream, subconscious, conscious (or awake) and unconscious (as in a coma). These states of consciousness are not what we are concerned with here.

Philosophers such as David Chalmers and Robert Forman view consciousness as a fundamental force of the universe, that exists everywhere and in everything. All living things have some form of consciousness and intelligence.

Besides consciousness emanating from us, the self being part of this source of consciousness, we are being acted upon by this conscious field. We ourselves are mostly space and electromagnetic energy and therefore have access to the energy that pervades the universe. Einstein's mathematical equation relating energy to mass and Quantum physics' duality of wave/particle lends scientific credence to this concept. Quantum physics in modern day science states that the ultimate principle of all matter is the same pure energy. The invisible electrical energy gives form as light or radiant heat.

Consciousness is thought to be at the heart of the process of evolution. The idea of a fundamental conscious force which is perceived as pervading the whole of reality is common to most indigenous groups. The Lakota Indians called it *wakan-tanka*, or spirit-energy. It is usually seen as an all-pervasive force or power, with no gender or personality. The Gaia theory describes Earth as a living system with human society as a part of that system. This shared system of consciousness is the fundamental connection between living beings. You are a drop in a mighty ocean as much as *"the mighty ocean in a drop,"* poetically stated by Rumi.

Originally neuroscientists had hoped that consciousness could be located in a specific area of the brain through MRI studies. Although it is said that *"consciousness emerges from the operations of the brain"* no evidence to date is available for the nature or process of consciousness.

The nebulous nature of consciousness is very much open to interpretation. Wikipedia defines consciousness as *"the fact of awareness by the mind of itself and the world,"* The consciousness I refer to embraces two elements: our subjective, inner self (including our thoughts, feelings and perceptions) and our awareness of the world and the cosmos (or what happens outside of self). It reflects Emmanuel Kant's *"the starry heavens above me and the moral law within me."* The third eye chakra or inner wisdom is how we access the truth within as well as without—the unity in duality.

INNER WORLD   OUTER WORLD

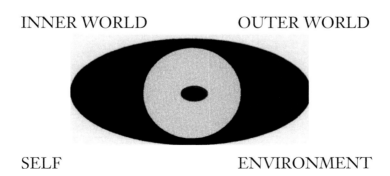

SELF   ENVIRONMENT

CONSCIOUSNESS

It is with the third eye or mystical, inner eye of consciousness that we can see oneself as part of a whole within the universe. These two (complex) petals of the sixth chakra hold the key to transformation. To be wholly human is to find the balance between the demands/pleasures of society and the requirements/yearnings of the inner life.

Chapter 29
THE SELF

Celebrate…..
Take a stand,
Declare yourself, sing I am
Boldly and with rejoicing
Not only to the stars at night
But to anyone anywhere
Without apologies or regrets.
　　　　—Gloria Burgess, "Song to Myself"

"Knowing others is intelligence; knowing yourself is true
wisdom. Mastering others is strength; mastering your-
self is true power."

　　　　　　　　　　　　—Lao Tzu

Many stories and myths have been written about the quest for
the "Holy Grail." The Holy Grail has been a coveted Christian
relic for centuries. The grail is most commonly identified as the
cup that Jesus drank from at the Last Supper and is supposedly

endowed with special powers. The Grail has also been used as a theme in fantasy, historical fiction and science fiction. King Arthur's knights quests after the Holy Grail.

The human being is constantly striving and seeking to find what life is all about. By turning inward to a journey of self-discovery, into the essence of one's own being, is to lead us to the "grail." The ultimate quest for the Holy Grail is the quest for self-empowerment and self-transformation.

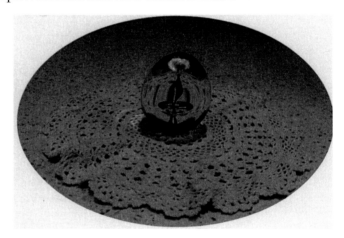

The Tao Te Ching states, *"This is true knowledge, to seek the Self as the true end of wisdom always."* This Self is sometimes called the "True Self," the "Observing Self," or the "Witness." The self is a central theme of many world religions. In Hindu philosophy, it is called the "atman" or essence and the goal of life is to realize the fundamental truth about oneself. Patañjali's Yoga-Sutra expresses it as *"union with one's real identity, after putting to rest all movements in the mind."*

The nature of "the self" has been expounded extensively by philosophers and psychologists right from the time of Aristotle. Inscribed in the stone at the Oracle of Delphi was the admonition *"know thyself."* Polonius, in Shakespeare's *Hamlet*, advises his son who is leaving for France and states, *"to thine own self be true."* Our need to know, explain and understand ourselves has continued throughout the ages. C. J. Jung, the great psychologist, posits that the Self is the total persona, which includes consciousness, the unconscious, and the ego. The Self is the totality of the whole psyche.

Jean-Paul Sartre's epiphany regarding Descartes statement, *"I think, therefore I am,"* realized that *"the consciousness that says 'I am' is not the consciousness that thinks,"* He therefore infers that the truer statement should be *"I am therefore I think."*

The self is the "I am"—the being that exists before thought or language. This self is the agent responsible for our thoughts and actions. The self is not a place or thing that can be found on the genetic code or though dissection of the brain and body. The self not a fixed body of matter, but is a field of energy and information, that is evolving as an ongoing process. "Self is a sea boundless and measureless." writes Kahlil Gibran.

This ongoing effort of self-understanding or finding the author or songwriter of one's life is the process of individuation. It involves the active pursuit of knowledge with self-exploration and autonomy of thought. Self-actualization is a continued process of growth and becoming; not a static state. It is a rugged path lined with blackberry bushes. We are pricked by its thorns even as we pick the sweet, luscious berries. As Aldous Huxley says, self-knowledge is painful and we often prefer to remain in a blissful state of ignorance.

Understanding of self unlocks the door to an inherent, vast potential. The process of individuation requires a desire to dig deep to know oneself and become more of what one is capable of becoming. It encompasses the basic three Rs: reflection, respect and responsibility. These three elements motivate the self to initiate specific behaviors and mental attitudes that are essential for psychological health and well-being.

The quest for the Holy Grail or authentic individuation requires reflection and internal dialogue. Jesus retreats up a high mountain where with deep reflection he was "transfigured." Buddha studied under the greatest spiritual teachers, lived a life of renunciation without finding the truth. It was when he retreated under the Bodhi tree and reflected on the nature of things that he gained "enlightenment."

> *"Knowing the self is enlightenment. To seek anything else is ignorance."*
>
> —Bhagavad Gita.

Aristotle speaks of the virtues of a contemplative life and Socrates held that the unexamined life is not worth living. The yoga sutras explain self-reflection as *"bringing one's awareness and one's thoughts within."* Christians propose the four steps of "Lectio Divina" which is to read, meditate, pray and contemplate. Eastern religions recommend transcendental meditation. It is a commitment to intentionally know oneself; to find our inner world, examining and experiencing self. Consciously closing one's mind processes to the sensory world to understand self is to surf the "Inner Net." Moving away from the activity of the mind and into the stillness, we tap into a vast realm of intelligence beyond thought and mind—an intrinsic, universal wisdom often alluded to as Sophia.

Self-reflection demands introspection and personal insight coupled with critical inquiry.

As we develop the ability to be the object of our own reflection we attain a higher level of consciousness. It liberates us from our emotions and makes us more thoughtful and a better person. By analyzing our life experiences there is less repetition of negative patterns in daily life. We reflect, not to wallow in our limitations or failures, but to creatively deal with them as resources for a full and better life.

Once we pose the pertinent questions, we find the inner resources to address it and interpret its relevance and its application. *"Who am I in the midst of all this thought traffic?"* says Rumi.

Mulling over questions such as "who am I and why am I here" honors the attempt to live one's life authentically, according to the needs of one's inner being and focus on what is really important in life. As we do so we develop a healthy respect for self.

The English dictionary defines self-respect as a proper regard for one's own dignity and integrity. Kant was the first major Western philosopher to put respect for persons, including oneself as a person, at the very center of moral theory.

It is impossible not to have a sense of reverence and awe for the human body. All our organ systems are delicately balanced, interrelated and synchronized. Our skeletal system forms the framework that houses our being. Our skin functions as a protective barrier and a thermostat. Our senses and emotions form the security system, and the endocrine glands regulate and fine tune all functions. Our muscular system allows for locomotion and activity. Our brain with its vast library, functions as the administrative office. Our heart motor supplies a river of nutrients and energy to the body. Our lungs like efficient bellows, ventilate, exchanging unwanted carbon dioxide for fresh oxygen. The kidneys, our central plumbing system, filter and purify blood and eliminate waste. The digestive system processes foods for the sustenance of all body cells and comes equipped with a built in clean up tract for elimination of waste. Remarkably, we sustainably pass these largesse to subsequent generations through our reproductive system. All these wondrous gifts are components of the human body without cost or effort on our part. Yet there is only one of us in all time and no two are alike. Combinations of form, feelings, perceptions and thought processes are uniquely individual. Compared to the cosmos, we are smaller than a grain of sand on the beach yet no less of a miracle of creation—the paradox of being insignificant and yet precious beyond measure.

Once we recognize our essential awesomeness we can give complete self-acceptance and respect, precisely as we are. We can also appreciate that the physical body is the chalice (holy grail) or receptacle for the self. Learning to be mindful and direct our attention inward we find the treasure within.

Organ systems may fail but the underlying self continues to be a resilient being in the face of adversity. Take Christopher Reeves or Steven Hawking for example. Their "self" is projected in amazing ways in spite of a great number of body system failures. There is a sense of wholeness independent of physical symptoms and impairments.

"Insist on yourself; never imitate. Your own gift you can offer with the cumulative force of a whole life's cultivation, but of the adopted talent of another, you have only an extemporaneous, half possession."
—Ralph Waldo Emerson

With respect and reverence comes the responsibility to care for self. We need to accept responsibility for our own life, our own experience and inner personal growth not because of religious or social mandates but because of data that supports this wisdom for health. Respecting ourselves we can take the responsibility and turn away from destructive patterns whether it is food, drugs, thoughts or words. Only when we better understand ourselves can we secure the relationship to the self that has so often eluded us. We may not achieve perfection but, with intent, can set our sights higher.

We can take the responsibility for our inner space and creatively turn tragic aspects of life to accomplishment. In *"The mature mind,"* Gene D. Cohen states that developing a healthy balance of inner resources reduces stress and increases sense of choice and control. We are responsible for finding inherent value and meaning in our ordinary, everyday life. It requires wrestling with, and coming to grips with our emotional and intellectual faculties. Personal development is based on growing and expanding our awareness. By accepting personal responsibility for our thoughts, perceptions and circumstances, we greatly enhance our power to change our life. With positive change comes a sense of wholeness, fulfilment and health.

> *"The art of being is … discovery and discernment of our inner world so we can connect with our true essence and remain virtuous to our sweet fragrant selves."*
> —Ali ibn Abi Talib.

Journaling the day's happenings, all our activities and efforts, accepting our shortcomings and limitations, can help us focus on what we need, to take care of ourselves. "What can I learn from this experience" and "what could I have done better" allows us the insight to make better decisions. Just as in the presence of light there is no darkness, self-awareness sheds light in our dark corners enabling us to be more conscious in times of difficulty. Living from our center in tune with the source within, is like a musician who experiences the music from within and explodes it outwardly. Finding self we find the music and the abundance of life. In "The power of Myth" Joseph Campbell posits that rather than a meaning for life, what we are seeking is the rapture of being alive—finding experiences that resonate with the core of our innermost being.

Medical Applications

Dan Siegel states that once we become aware of our *mental processes and patterns* we are attuned to ourselves and become enabled to change and make better, healthier choices.

Staying stuck in thoughts and emotions we remain a victim of the mind. A shift in consciousness leads to a cascade of healing responses and promotes healing from within. Psychotherapy uses these principles in different ways to effect a change in behavior and mood.

Meditative Exercise

Thoreau, in order to discover life's true essential needs, built his hermitage on the lake and inspired the world. Incessant mental noise and physical activity prevents us from finding that realm of inner stillness. Stillness is a refreshing way to rejuvenate and find fresh perspective. When inwardly quiet, the voice of wisdom, or Sophia, speaks.

Find a quiet place free from distraction. Keep the breath soft; breathing in and breathing out feel the waves of relaxation. Access the infinite source of wisdom by going into the stillness, or the space between thought.

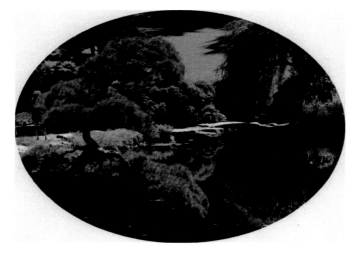

Bainbridge WA

It is natural for the mind to revert to its mindless, repetitive, mental chatter. By bringing back the wandering mind we strengthen the power of attention and focus; we build the muscle of attention. As your thoughts float by, watch the thinker and dissociate from your thoughts. You will feel a conscious presence of your essential self, deeper than the floating thoughts or mind.

Develop a healthy relationship with this precious self; accessing it often. Realize the Holy Grail brimming with the treasure of self. Make every day of your life a celebration, sculpting your beautiful life one stroke at a time.

Chapter 30
THE ENVIRONMENT

"Radiate boundless love towards the entire world—above, below, and across—unhindered, without ill will, without enmity."
—The Buddha, *The Metta Sutra*

"My brother asked the birds to forgive him: that sounds senseless, but it is right; for all is like an ocean, all is flowing and blending; a touch in one place sets up movement at the other end of the earth."
—Fyodor Dostoyevsky, *Brothers Karmazov*

The first environment we are exposed to is the womb. Knowing what we know about genetics and epigenetics, we can appreciate that the prenatal environment plays a greater role in the development of the fetus than previously understood. Fetal nerve receptors respond to molecular signals as well as energy signals. Hence fetal growth and development can be altered by maternal nutrition, as well as thoughts and emotions. This should give food for thought for all prospective parents.

We have always known that infants imitate what they see. Scientists have discovered that there are neurons in an animal that fire both when the animal acts as well as when the animal observes the same action performed by another. They call this mirror neurons. In humans this function probably involves much more complex circuits involving the insula and superior temporal regions, as well as aspects of the prefrontal cortex. This process of influencing and being influenced by others is referred to as *limbic regulation*. A related term is "limbic resonance" which is an interpersonal harmony that arises from connecting with another. Resonance is a sympathetic vibration between two elements, such as a sound, bell or musical tone that allows them to synchronize with a new harmony.

Besides responding to actions that we observe in others, these mirror neuron circuits are possibly responsible for a myriad of other sophisticated human behavior and thought processes. It allows us to feel what others are experiencing, instinctively understand their intentions and appreciate and learn from their actions.

As we grow, our environment expands to the family home, followed by institutions of learning and place of work. The health of the family determines the health of the child and ultimately the health of the world. Our systems synchronize with one another with profound implications for lifelong emotional health. By entering the emotional space of the other, we stimulate resonance circuits in unconscious ways. The pleasure hormone oxytocin is released when we are in contact with another in a positive relationship. Our brains are intensely social and relationships have a huge impact on nervous system and brain chemistry from the earliest days of our lives. Longing for connection is a basic human drive drawing one person to another.

Our lives have meaning, only in relationship to the other and to the external world. A sense of social purpose and attention to the well-being of others serves to grow the mind. The support and opportunities offered by others nourish us. Being needed boosts our own sense of worth and happiness; and as we value and enjoy others, we radiate joy.

The Heart Math Research Institute has shown that the electromagnetic field of the heart can be measured from two to three meters away from the body. They discovered that someone with a coherent heart rhythm has a positive effect on other people in close proximity. Coherence implies order and harmony. The energy of this harmony or serenity transfers from one person to another. Positive interpersonal resonance can be compared to the strings of a violin vibrating together in harmony. Each string with its own pure note; the whole forming one harmonious chord, richer than a string on its own. We are part of the whole and are interdependent on each other irrespective of race, nationality or creed.

By the same token, disharmony or anger from one can influence reciprocal feelings in another. Rebel rousers use this emotional contagion to rile up crowds.

Wordless transfer of information can occur between minds at a distance. We only have to consider the magic of iPhones and wireless computers to grasp this concept with its potential. We have yet to explore, understand and harness this power.

Besides affecting the mental and emotional states of others, resonance can occur with all of creation. Man is a microcosm that mirrors the larger macrocosm. The Eastern cultures have had an appreciation of this consciousness at least as early as the sixth century BCE as determined by the I Ching and the Upanishads. According to Eastern thought, the five elements, the environmental factors of wood, fire, earth, metal and water that are part of the macrocosm equally apply to the human microcosm. This five element concept is used to explain a wide array of phenomena, linking cosmic cycles to internal organs and to the properties of foods and medicinal drugs.

Human health is intrinsically connected to planet health. Being responsible for and increasing our personal vibration to earth's resonance is reflected in improved personal health and happiness. We can directly affect the physical world through our conscious awareness and intentionally shape the future of the world we live in.

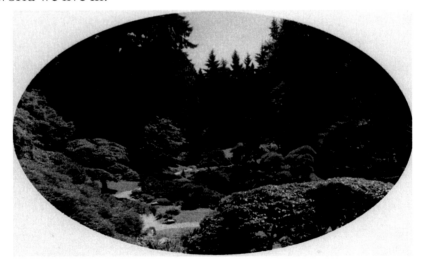

There is no line of separation as we are one with the whole limitless boundary of the universe. Every dew drop on a spider's web contains the reflection of every other dew drop and its reflections, ad infinitum. Every whole has a relationship with and is a part of a greater whole. This concept is illustrated by the concept of Indra's net. According to Hindu myth, the Vedic god Indra has a net hanging over his palace at mount Meru and spread across the vast expanse of space. At every knot of the net is a multifaceted jewel that reflects all the other jewels; every person is intimately connected with all in the universe. Each person has their own place within the net yet we all reflect and influence each other. This is what interconnectedness means. We shape the universe as much as the universe shapes us.

"The wild geese do not intend to cast their reflection.
The water has no mind to receive their image"
—Zen poet

The Gaia hypothesis is an approach to understand our world as a global ecosystem. Our planet is shaped with an optimal environment for life, and life maintains the stability of the natural environment. Trees and rocks and rivers are to this world the bones and blood streams of the body. All of creation must be valued as part of nature. We share the same sun, moon and planets; we breathe the same air. Plants consciously turn their leaves to the sun and send their roots to water. Mankind basks in the sun and dies without water. The earth sustains us, and it is our mandatory responsibility to nurture and take care of mother earth.

According to Hindu doctrine, Creation was set in motion by the universal vibration represented by the sound "aum." AUM symbolizes the infinite ultimate reality and the entire universe. Repeating this sacred sound as a mantra or prayer, with the correct intonation, is said to bring awareness to all that is; resonating the center of one's being with cosmic vibration.

There is a one-ness of man and the cosmos. Carl Sagan elaborates this by saying that "the cosmos is within us; we are made of star stuff." *Cosmos: A Personal Voyage* (wikiquote).

Since ancient times man has had an attraction to, and curiosity of, the "heavens." The Babylonians predicted the weather through recognition of cloud patterns and stars. The wise men in the bible "read" the heavens and were led to the baby Jesus. We now use measurable qualities of the atmosphere such as rain, wind, humidity, temperature and pressure for important forecasts to protect life and property. Networks of seismographs facilitate the monitoring and analysis of global earthquakes and other sources of seismic activity. Our exploration and curiosity has progressed to the utilization of wind power and solar energy.

Independent lines of research show that people are indeed affected by Earth's energetic environment and that the universe is very much interconnected and coherent. Ongoing research is supporting the existence of a global information field of consciousness that is common to all living systems. Carl Sagan in the TV series *Cosmos:A Personal Voyage* states *"we have found that scientific laws pervade all of nature; that the same rules apply on Earth as in the skies; that we can find a resonance, a harmony between the way we think and the way the world works."* Repeating patterns in nature are the natural laws of the cosmos. Every cell and biological circuit in our body is endowed with this conscious force of solar and cosmic origins. Solar and Earth's magnetic fields affect human nervous system functioning, just as surely as surface ocean tides rise and fall predictably, due to changes in gravitational forces originating from the Moon and the Sun. Our thoughts and lives affects the cosmic expression and flow as much as the shape of the shoreline and the ocean floor changes the flow of tides.

This interactive, synchronized relationship with the solar systems is seen in numerous physiological patterns in humans. Our bodies wake up with the sun and sleep with its setting. The menstrual cycle follows a lunar month. We hunker down in winter and spring after the equinox.

Just three centuries ago man believed that the earth was the center of the universe. Then Galileo through his telescope, observed that the earth was not central to the universe and that we moved around the sun. Close observation of what exists was brought to awareness and is now part of common knowledge. The universe has far more secrets to share than ever dreamed of, and is worthy of our curiosity and exploration. *"Our future depends powerfully on how well we understand this cosmos in which we float like a mote of dust in the morning sky."*—Carl Sagan, *Cosmos* (Wikiquote LCC QB44.2.S235).

Medical Applications

Relationships heal and repair wounded minds. Meaningful connections with others have a greater positive impact on the incidence of illness and premature death than diet, genetics, drugs or medical intervention. A healthy social network is associated with lower blood pressure and reduces the risk of heart attacks and strokes. Positive social relationships reduce stress. Stress hormones impair the immune system, burden the heart and increase risk for anxiety and depression.

People with at least three to four intimate contacts and strong healthy social networks live longer, deal better with stress and have healthier endocrine, cardiovascular and immune systems. It is through our personal connection to a place and people within, that we gain a sense of belonging, and create memories to give significance and meaning to our life.

The Global Coherence Initiative (GCI) is a project based on the hypothesis that when enough individuals and social groups increase their coherence, authentic compassion and caring will increase globally through the power of collective intention and consciousness. GCI is working in concert with other initiatives to realize this potential to address society's significant social, environmental, and economic problems. The "mood" of the planet needs to change from violence, war and terror to peace and tranquility.

Environments designed with a sense of harmony and congruence enhance human happiness. Sustainable urban design with a focus on functionality, social equity and beauty allows society to function better as a whole. Reducing light and noise pollution and increasing opportunities for social interaction, enhances livability for its inhabitants. Safe self-contained communities surrounded by nature promotes stress-free environments.

The field of sustainable, environmental health and protection, focused on the natural and built environments, is gaining ground in popularity. It addresses climate change, ecosystem degradation, species extinctions, and biodiversity losses that threaten human health on local, regional, and global scales. It is targeted towards preventing disease and creating supportive environments for the benefit of human health, through qualitative research methods and behavioral change interventions.

We can each do our part in keeping our own personal environment healthy, reflecting compassion, and caring for this precious Earth.

Meditative Exercise

Amongst the myriad planets, ours is the one chosen to host all of life and its wonders as far as we know. We cannot but marvel at the awesomeness of our planet whatever we believe its origins to be. Quoting Emerson, *"If there were but one starlit night a year everyone on the planet would stop to herald the annual pageant of light."*

Take nature walks with slow deliberate steps. As you walk let your mind quieten. Synchronise your steps with your breath. The mind is the most still during the pause between the inhalation and the exhalation.

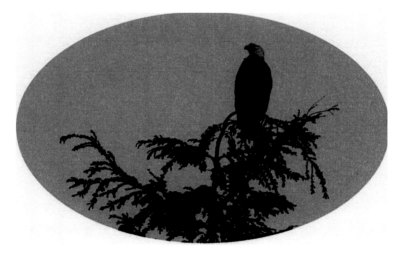

Look for and appreciate the majesty and grandeur of experiences everywhere around you: the growth of plants and flowers; birds and animals in the wild, cherry blossoms and sparkling snowcapped mountains; a glorious sunset; the serenity of a full moon.

Recollect the three R's from the last chapter. *Reflect* on who you are and how you are connected to family, community, universe and the cosmos. *Respect* nature, its rhythms and the changes of the seasons that enrich the fabric of daily living. Take personal *responsibility* for creating and supporting a healthy community, nation and world, right where you are. Strive to achieve *resonance* (the fourth R) with all of creation.

Reflection and meditation lead the way to awareness and understanding.

CHAKRA 7

THE CROWN CHAKRA
THOUSAND PETALS OF INTEGRATION

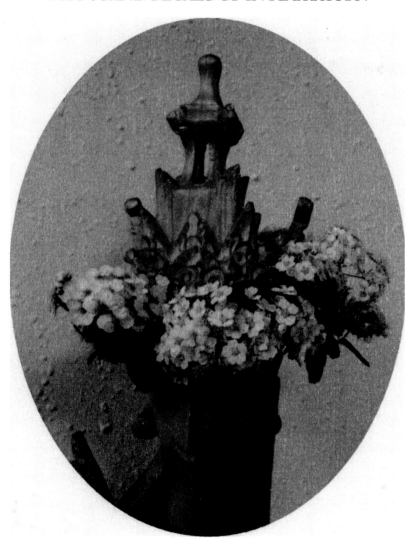

Chapter 31
A THOUSAND PETALS OF INTEGRATION

"May you have enough happiness to make you sweet, enough trials to make you strong, enough sorrow to keep you human and enough hope to make you happy. Be really whole and all things will come to you."

—Lao Tzu

The seventh chakra, or the crown chakra, is the merging of all chakras just as its color, white, is the presence of the entire spectrum of visible light. In the Bible, light was created immediately after the heavens and the earth. White, in Western culture, is the color most often associated with new beginnings. White is commonly associated with innocence, perfection, and purity, being worn for auspicious occasions such as baptism, first communion, and as bridal apparel. People with positive near death experiences report sudden immersion in a powerful white light with a sense of peace, well-being, unconditional love, and acceptance.

Traditionally the crown chakra is said to be the source of enlightenment with the realization that everything is connected at a fundamental level. This chakra is depicted as the 1,000 petals of a lotus flower opening to allow human flourishing or eudaimonia. A comparable Inuit word is *"Nuannaarpoq,"* meaning *"the extravagant pleasure in being alive."* But what human flourishing really is, depending on who one asks, varies from wealth and power to leading a healthy, simple life. The road to achieve this goal is also highly variable.

From the time of Socrates, there has been a consensus that all people thirst for health and happiness. To Socrates, moral virtue is the most important good and argues that life is not worth living if the soul is ruined by wrongdoing. Plato argues for being a just person whose soul is ordered and harmonious. Lack of inner harmony and unity hinders the achievement of eudaimonia. For Aristotle, eudaimonia is the attainment of excellence in reason and the highest good, attained for its own sake.

We chase happiness with extrinsic goals of money, image and status. Sadly, we fill our lives with busyness and distractions to temporarily release us from our restless longings and needs. We experiment with drugs to kill boredom, self-doubt, loneliness, and anxiety.

The Fourth King of Bhutan, in the 1970s, coined the term Gross National Happiness (GNH) to measure the health of his country rather than Gross Domestic Product (GDP) which reflects the economic value of a nation. The term implies a comprehensive, holistic picture of the happiness of Bhutanese beyond material fulfilment and physical well-being. The GNH philosophy considers that all aspects of life contribute to the human potential to achieve true happiness.

According to Buddhist teaching, happiness is freedom from want, and suffering is unfulfilled desire. The happiest of people don't necessarily have all of everything but they make the most of what they have.

Maslow states that for greater wholeness as a human being, all needs should be fulfilled. He formulated a hierarchy of needs that has since been modified from a five step to an eight-stage model. His model is a pyramid moving from the lowest biological and physiological needs to the highest cognitive, aesthetic and transcendent needs that we must satisfy in turn. However, we have seen that a homeless person can show compassion to another fellow being and have a complex philosophy of life in spite of his basic needs not being met.

I would posit that human behavior is tied in to all the chakras in a holistic, integrated way. With the holistic chakra system formulated here, a nesting of needs rather than a pyramid or hierarchy of needs is proposed. All needs (chakras) have the same emphasis and each is contained in the other; just as white contains all the wavelengths of visible light at approximately equal intensities. Although from an evolutionary standpoint the higher chakras developed at a later stage and is more complex in function, each supports and strengthens the other. Another analogy is to see the chakras connected as an ever widening spiral. Each turn of the spiral continuous with the ones before.

By integration of all the chakras, we can strive for personal growth. We can understand life at a deeper level to achieve Eudaimonia; a life that pulsates in exquisite harmony. We perform better when thoughts, emotions, values and goals are in balance, with time for rest, play, relationships and daily tasks.

In 2014, the British National Health Service began recommending a five step plan for living meaningful lives and mental well-being. The five steps, in a nutshell, are: (1) Connection with community and family; (2) Physical exercise; (3) Lifelong learning;

(4) Giving to others; (5) Mindfulness of the world around. Integration of the seven chakras incorporates and expands on these five steps.

Health and happiness and wholeness is about being in harmony and at peace with oneself even when faced with physical or emotional ailments, just as much as a tree can thrive with a parasitic vine trailing up its trunk or after a branch is severed. A person dying of cancer or terminal illness can still be a healthy person. Health is not just the absence of disease; health comes from within. Health and wholeness is about understanding all our chakras and accepting and integrating all aspects of our humanity. Eudaimonia is when we maximize and utilize all the colors of the chakras.

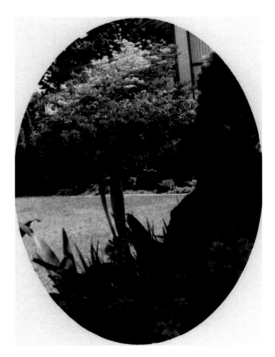

Like facets of a diamond each chakra reflects an inseparable aspect of the whole. Polishing one facet enhances the other facets of the jewel. By integrating the chakras, the end result becomes greater than the sum of all. The 1000 petals of the crown chakra represents abundance.

> *"And all these things shall be added unto you."*
> —Matthew 6:33 kjv

Because of improved health care and public health measures, the average US life expectancy was seventy-nine years in 2012, up from thirty years in the year 1600. However, the Commonwealth Fund, a research organization for better health practices, shows that the U.S. spends more on health care (seventeen percent of GDP) than any other high-income countries; but with poorer outcomes, a greater prevalence of chronic conditions and a shorter life expectancy. There is also a greater use of medical technology and pharmaceuticals with its accompanying high costs. U.S. spending on social services made up a relatively small share of the economy relative to other countries. Not enough emphasis is being given to other health parameters such as mental and emotional health, ethics and values, self-esteem, and expression. A holistic approach incorporating all aspects of life as outlined by the seven chakras in this book would be a cost-effective way to improve patients' health and reduce the dependence on medical technology and pharmaceuticals. Denmark has taken baby steps to achieve this by offering free education, health care and housing. Expanding education to include education for living not just education to make a living, will make for a better and healthier society.

Flying low under a starlit night we see the myriad city lights interconnected by an electrical power source. Electrical utility providers found it more efficient and cost effective to interconnect their transmission systems through the recently developed 'smart grid'—which is the electrical grid enhanced by information technology. The smart grid turns the electrical grid, through which power is generated and transmitted, into an intelligent network or mesh whose nodes are all connected to each other. By this power of integration, efficiency and productivity are maximized. There is often more than one path between a source and its destination in the network to allow for alternate pathways.

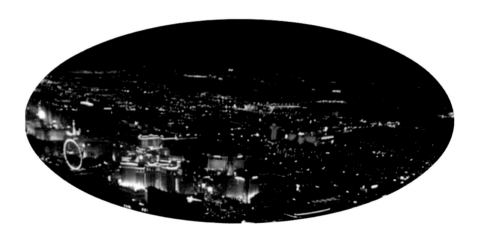

The human body functions in a similar manner with its integrated systems in the brain, nerves and organs. Our maximum potential and happiness is when there is harmony and balance with the chakras interconnected and integrated. Recognizing this, we can strive for integration for our own happiness and well-being.

Integration is the act of bringing together smaller varying components into a single comprehensive system that functions as one. We can think of integration as the synchronization of mental and bodily processes, the environment and all that is, over time. Thus, integration can be graphically visualized as a three dimensional model of horizontal, vertical and time/space coordinates. This is comparable to a compressed version of Maslow's hierarchy of needs and Alderfer's Existence, Relatedness and Growth (ERG) theory. It is closely allied with the current Dalai Lama's teaching of knowledge, love and action. The three dimensions are expanded on in the next chapter.

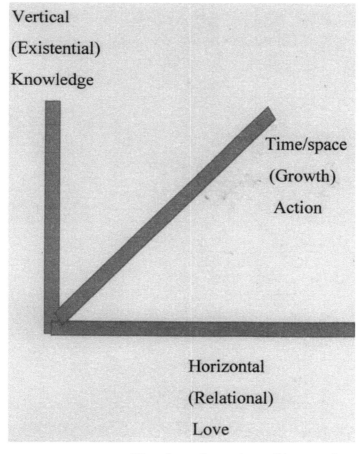

Vertical

(Existential)

Knowledge

Time/space

(Growth)

Action

Horizontal

(Relational)

Love

The three dimensions of integration

Chapter 32
THE THREE DIMENSIONS

"This is how to contemplate our conditioned existence in this fleeting world: Like a tiny drop of dew, or a bubble floating in a stream; Like a flash of lightning in a summer cloud, Or a flickering lamp, an illusion, a phantom, or a dream."

—Diamond Sutra

"Few will have the greatness to bend history itself; but each of us can work to change a small portion of events, and the total of those acts will be written in the history of this generation."

—Robert F. Kennedy

Vertical Integration

Awakening essentially is a development in consciousness often depicted as a snake. The snake is metaphorically associated with rebirth or renewal. The shedding of its old skin represents the release of old ways into rebirth and new beginnings. The Aztecs worshipped Quetzalcoatl, the Feathered Serpent, an amalgamation of the magnificent green-plumed quetzal bird and the snake, symbolizing knowledge, learning and renewal.

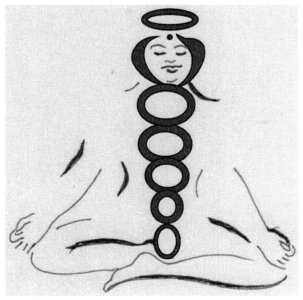

In Vedic literature, the serpent signifies "kundalini rising" or the "awakening of the kundalini," which means being aware of and developing consciousness or inner knowledge. In the chakra system the serpent forms loops around the energy centers. The looped serpent on either side of the energy centers can be thought to represent the vertical integration of the chakras. By integrating our understanding of ourselves our consciousness expands and we embark on new beginnings. Remaining focused on our lower chakras we persist in delusion, ignorance, and stagnate in frivolous matters. As we integrate and incorporate every aspect of the six chakras in our daily life we bring more balance and fullness to our lives. We become more fully who we were meant to be.

Anatomically, the serpents around the energy centers can be viewed as the vagus nerve. The vagus nerve is the longest nerve in the body that starts in the brain and travels down to the pelvic organs. Like the snake it slithers downward on its path with branches to the nerve plexuses and cross fibers to the opposite side. With its multiple elements of motor, sensory, sympathetic and parasympathetic nerve fibers, it integrates all the functions of body that occur without need for conscious control. Nature, it appears, recognizes and provides for integration. A healthy vagal tone, with an optimal firing rate of the sympathetic/parasympathetic fibers, promotes harmony between enthusiasm and relaxation. It orchestrates a natural coherence for the digestive, cardiovascular, neurological, reproductive, and immune repair mechanisms of the body. It has been found that meditative practices stimulate and strengthens the vagus nerve resulting in health benefits to all the organ systems.

Knowledge, awareness and application of the full totality of our existence lead to optimal health. Eating too much, too little, irregular meals or the wrong foods are factors that lead to ill health. What we put in our bodies gets metabolized and forms the structure of our cells. Overuse, under use or wrongful use of our musculature leads to pain and dysfunction of muscles and joints. Negative thoughts and destructive emotions affect every cell of our bodies and wreak havoc over time. Not living in alignment with our values creates an internal conflict that is toxic to cells. Stifling our voices of individuality and creativity we harbor discontent and disease.

Understanding our place in the universe we synchronize inner and outer being. Integration and utilization of all our chakras enhances our minds and improves physical, emotional, intellectual and psychological capabilities. Claiming this knowledge and making it our own, we can intentionally invite changes in thought patterns, habits and conduct to sustain health related behaviors. Working on ourselves, incorporating all the chakras, sets us on a path to realize our full potential.

Horizontal Integration

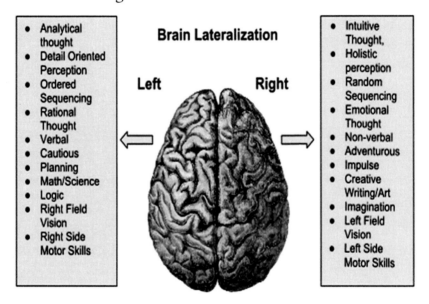

Author, Chickens are so cute
https://creativecommons.org

The body also naturally accommodates horizontal integration. The brain is divided into the right and left cerebral hemispheres. The two halves are connected by the corpus callosum. The corpus callosum facilitates communication between the two sides of the brain and transfers motor, sensory, and cognitive information between the brain hemispheres. Cross connections create a richer, more vivid experience because the brain is drawing on a broader palette of resources for the task. The intuitive and non-verbal brain skills in the right complements the logical left brain. The memory of an event through the left brain is infused with meaning by the feelings from the right brain. The words of a song from the left brain are harmonized by the right brain.

Our right and left hemispheres of the brain control the contralateral side of our bodies. The right hemisphere processes and controls our left side while the left hemisphere controls and processes the right side. Activating the power of both hemispheres we have more assets and variability of function.

Going beyond the physical body, horizontal integration encompasses the love, friendship and joy that make life worth living through relationships. Horizontal integration can be seen in many aspects of our life; in government, language, religion, fashion, sports, cuisine, music and dance. An idea or skill from elsewhere is integrated, merging with what is and made anew.

Jackie Robinson broke the color bar to be the first African American to play in Major League Baseball and set the stage for integration of blacks into the sporting arena. The beauty of integration is captured by the uniquely American art form of Jazz. Its musical give-and-take use of improvisation, blends together Ragtime, syncopated spirituals, marching band music, and the soulful Blues. The ethnic melting pot of Spanish, French, and African and Cuban influences present in New Orleans was the breeding ground for zydeco and calypso. African and Latin cultures hybridized their dance to evolve samba, salsa, and cumbia. Buddhism, originating in India, has been incorporated into aspects of Shintoism in Japan to form Zen Buddhism.

Integration does not mean forced assimilation as is often the case in countries where there is imperial power. Christianity and Catholicism was forced on indigents by conquering nations, raping their culture. By the same token, America's concept of democracy should not be forcibly imposed on countries not ready for or open to these ideas.

The earliest interpretations on existential questions were mythical in nature. History, and details surrounding events, change over time as stories are retold. Jorge Luis Borges expresses this as a truth fundamental to all religions. He states that legends are created to explain the complex realities of life and its mysteries; oral language being inadequate. These stories become embellished and embedded in societies all over the world over time, unintentionally perpetuating these false tales.

Reviewing the major religions of the world we see that The Abrahamic traditions emphasize a relationship to "God." The Hindu religion focuses on the multiple faces of the Creator and the invisible net that connects all mankind. Hinduism (as well as ancient Greeks) see gods and goddesses in every aspect of life honoring the holiness in all we do. The Native American, Australian, and Maori cultures revere the land and all its creatures, finding divinity in all living things. The Baha'i Faith emphasizes spiritual growth and service to humanity. Sikhs balance their moral and spiritual values with the quest for knowledge, promoting a life of peace, equality and positive action. Buddhists point to the inward journey and relationship to self. No religion has the monopoly on truth or morality. Gandhi describes the different religions as beautiful flowers from the same garden, or branches from the same tree.

The meaning of life ultimately boils down to how we integrate our religious/spiritual perspectives in our ordinary daily human existence. By opening our minds we can assimilate what is appealing in the beliefs of others and incorporate those aspects into our own belief systems. By so doing, we weave a rich fabric of meaning and holism into our lives. Personal freedom and enlightenment comes from integrating the vitality that is responsible for the creation of life and not from creeds or dogma.

Time/Space Integration

We see patterns across time throughout the history of civilization. Studying these patterns, we see that evolution and revelation go hand in hand. Our lives need to be put in perspective as a process in time; the past continuous with the present and the future. Artistically, integrating past, present and future as a continuum, Kehinde Wiley, a New York artist, has taken an ordinary black person from the streets and elevated them in a grand portraiture in the style of the eighteenth century with elaborate background tapestry, framing them for the pleasure of future generations.

The elaborate tombs of ancient Egypt and the catacombs of Rome bear witness to the reverence for those who have gone before. Culturally, the day of the dead, or *"dia de los muertos,"* in Mexico; "all saints day" in catholic communities; and ancestral worship in eastern cultures, celebrate the connection of the past with the living. Celebrations and rituals foster hope by promising a brighter future in the life hereafter.

In our individual lives we cannot divorce the events of the past from our existence. Neither can we ignore the future for ourselves and generations to come. But the present is the reality of our lives. Every day we can be open to Kairos, a Greek word denoting the opportune and decisive moment, period or season, when conditions are right for accomplishment. Like a glass blower we need to know just when to blow and when to cool our molten work of art. Our lives are but a moment in time and time but a moment of our lives.

The brain, like an idling locomotive, exhibits a resting network pattern of activity even when asleep. This baseline "noise" of intrinsic electrical activity within neuronal networks adds variability and an expanded palette to the neural response. Research suggests that "noise" increases with age and is a sign of greater complexity and integration in the brain. Thoughts, images, feelings and experiences, synchronize better with a coherent brain pattern. Older adults utilize the left and right hippocampi more so than the young who use the left hippocampus primarily. We become more complete as we grow. The child remains in blissful acceptance of the immediate with ignorance of all else. Coherence and variability in brain noise is shown to be enhanced with meditative practices resulting in improved cognitive functions.

Each lifespan stretches over time with bountiful treasures. Joseph Campbell's *Hero's Journey* chronicles the hero's return home with knowledge and wisdom acquired on the journey. We can learn to embrace the deepening wisdom, judgement and perspective through expanding consciousness and life experiences as we age.

We do not have to accept that our memory will inevitably decline in old age. It is often our own belief creating exactly what we fear. As we age consciously we become more authentically true to self, aware of new capabilities and gifts.

The Global Peace Index (GPI) is the brain child of Steve Killelea, the Australian philanthropist. The GPI measures global peace using three broad motifs: safety and security in society, domestic and international conflict, and the degree of militarization. The study, not surprisingly, shows that in more peaceful countries there is greater levels of transparency of government and lower corruption rates. The study draws attention to the huge resources squandered in violence and conflict and the senseless loss of precious lives. The money wasted in wars, incarcerations, and weapons could be better used to ending poverty, promoting education, and protecting the environment. Japan and Germany, once aggressors, now rank eighth and sixteenth out of 162, respectively on the peace index scale whereas the US ranks at ninety-four. We can learn from the over-arching story lines of history; the fall of the Roman Empire, the British Empire and Japanese and Chinese dynasties and the Vietnam and Iraq wars, to name a few. The collapse of empires can be shown in large part to be due to greed, corruption and social inequities. The lust for power, wealth and prestige discounts and disregards the needs of individuals. We need to take heed lest America cascades down this harrowing path to self-destruct. With its position of power and vast resources, the United States of America has an awesome potential to create peace by integrating cooperative, social relationships with the rest of the world; not by dominance and high-handed supremacy.

With advances in transportation and mobile media, cities and countries are tied closer in time and space. Society is becoming progressively complex and at the same time increasingly interdependent. We are no longer bounded by our locality but have social and economic ties globally. It is imperative that we work towards peaceful coexistence and collaboration.

With scientific advances we often falsely believe that the nature of reality is fully understood. However there has not been a satisfactory answer for many of the phenomena that we experience. For example the simultaneous scientific ideas or creative works by individuals living at different times and places or synchronistic happenings.

Quantum physics is attempting to answer these questions and to bring more understanding especially regarding space and locality. Nonlocality describes the apparent ability of particles to instantaneously know about each other's state, even when separated by large distances. Particles that interact with each other become permanently interrelated, or dependent on each other's states and properties. We are finding that quantum nonlocality is a property of the universe that is intrinsic to nature. At our tiniest, subatomic level we are all one inseparable network of Life. People, like particles described in quantum physics, may have instantaneous connections across distance. This is analogous to virtual cloud computing that enables users to access systems and share resources instantaneously using a web browser regardless of their location or what device they use.

With this knowledge we look toward a greater understanding of non-locality in remote healing and energy medicine. We have a long way to go to understand just how remote healing actually works. Apparently distance healing by intention is transmitted by an as yet unknown energy signal, which warps space-time for instantaneous connection. New studies are actively being undertaken all over the world to explore this new frontier.

Medical Applications

What we have done to our bodies, over time, eventually reaches a tipping point and manifests as ill health and may continue on as chronic illness. Unwholesome foods, tobacco, drugs and alcohol, as well as toxic emotions eventually takes its toll. The natural intelligence of the human body allows healing given time and the right conditions.

People with a stronger vagus response apparently recover more quickly after stress, injury, or illness. Neurosurgeon Kevin Tracey was the first to prove that stimulating the vagus nerve reduces inflammation. People with rheumatoid arthritis have shown improvement, and even remission, using electronic implants to stimulate the vagus nerve. This mode of therapy has been used to treat people with epilepsy and depression. Bioelectronics may be the future of medicine to treat illness with fewer medications and fewer side effects. Meditation and biofeedback can stimulate the vagus nerve to reap the health benefits without surgery.

Baseline brain 'Noise' levels increase in a chaotic manner with disorders such as schizophrenia and decrease with diseases such as Alzheimer's where memory, ideas, creativity and thoughts flatten out. By engaging in healthy, stimulating activities, we can maintain a healthy noise level in the brain and not accept the mental decline of aging as inevitable.

Meditative Exercise

The act of meditation and contemplation suppresses the interference of the thinking mind and allows true knowledge to surface. *"Be still and know."*

Be mindful of your breath, your senses and your environment. Reflect where you came from and the path of your personal development.

Construct your individual timeline chart chronicling the major themes and influences in your life. Consider positive and negative experiences, as well as life-transforming events. Allow the flourishing that comes with the evolution and the revelation of holistic living. Piece together the narrative of your life finding meaning and direction. See that there has been a time for everything *"and a time for every purpose."*

There is still that open road ahead of you. Set your compass to attain the highest limits of possibility that is right for you. Create the life you dream of and not stagnate in a life you don't want. Don't let precious moments of your life go by untouched or unused.

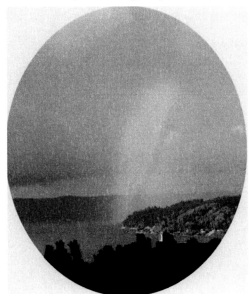

Be open to the rainbow of the chakras to experience the wonder and mystery of life.

"Life is not about how to survive the storm but how to dance in the rain.

—Anon

Life is short, ...Sail away from the safe harbor. Catch the trade winds in your sails. Explore. Dream. Discover."

—Mark Twain

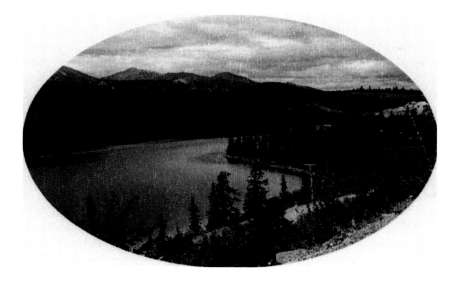

Allow the evolution and flourishing that comes with the revelations of holistic living.

And lastly to quote Forrest Gump's mama, the absolute authority:

LIFE
      IS
            LIKE
                  A
                       BOX
                              OF
                                      CHOCOLATES…

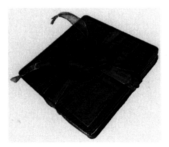

FURTHER READING

1. *How to Eat Healthy; Nutrition 101*
   10 Tips To Healthy Eating
   Cleveland Clinic, International Food Information Council
   Foundation, 1994
2. Frank Netter, MD—*Atlas of Human Anatomy*, Novartis
   Second Edition, 1997
3. Robin Fox—*Food and Eating: An Anthropological Perspective*,
   Pub. SIRC
4. Max Neuberger—*History of Medicine*, Oxford Press, 1910
5. Hippocrates—Encyclopedia Britannica, Nov. 1997
6. Carolyn Myss, Ph.D.—*Anatomy of the Spirit, The Seven Stages*, Harmony Books of Power and Healing, NY, 1996
7. Institute of Medicine Report—2013
8. Robert A Johnson—*We: Understanding the Psychology of Romantic Love*, Harper Collins, 1983
9. Robert A Johnson and Jerry M Ruhl, Ph.D.—*Living Your Unlived Life*, Jeremy P Tarcher, Penguin, 2007
10. Thich Nhat Hanh—*The Wisdom of Thich Nhat Hanh*, One Spirit Beacon and Parallax Press, 2007

11. Deepak Chopra—*Ageless Body Timeless Mind; The Quantum Alternative to Growing Old*, Harmony Books, 1993

12. Meg Lundstrom—*What To Do When You Can't Decide*, Sounds True Inc., Boulder, Colorado, 2010

13. Barrie Davenport—*The 52 Week Life Passion Project*, Blue Elephant Press, 2012

14. Elaine Fox—*Rainy Brain Sunny Brain*, Basic Books, 2012

15. Frederick M Hudson—*The Adult Years*, Jossey Bass Publishing

16. Paul Bloom—*How Pleasure Works*, WW Norton and Co

17. Elaine Stenger—*Dancing in the Rain*, Bilton House Publishing, 2010

18. Thomas Armstrong, Ph.D.—*The Human Oddyssey, Navigating the 12 Stages of Life*, Sterling Publishing, NY, London, 2007

19. Andrew Newburg—*The Mystical Mind Eugene d' Aquili and Probing the Biology of Religious Experience*, Fortress Press, 1999

20. Thomas Moore—*A Religion of One's Own*, Gotham Books, Penguin Pub, NY, 2014

21. Jonah Lehrer—*How We Decide*, Houghton Miflin Harcourt, NY, 2009

22. Malcolm Waters—*Daniel Bell*, Routledge, 1996

23. David Tacey—*How to Read Jung*, W. W. Norton & Co., 2006

24. Larry Dossey—*Healing Words*, Harper Collins, 1994

25. Eckhart Tolle—*The Power of Now*, Namaste Publishing, 1997

26. Amit Goswami, Ph.D.—*The Self Aware Universe*, Tarcher Putnam, 1995

27. Deepak Chopra—*The Path to Love*, Harmony Books, 1997
28. Dennis Coon—*Essentials of Psychology*, West Publishing Co., 1991
29. Anil Seth—*30 Second Brain*, Metro Books, NY, 2014
30. Richard Moss, MD—*The Mandala of Being*, New World Library, 2007

Acknowledgements

With humble gratitude I acknowledge the large part played by the University of Bastyr, Kenmore, Washington, in setting me on a journey of self-discovery. The Spirituality and Medicine course unfurled the tight bud of my mind and allowed the flowering. I continue in my search for authenticity, appreciating life and its many interfaces. I give credit to the muse that flowed through my hollow bones for the completion of this project.

I wish to thank all my fellow writers who have shared their inspiring memoirs and critiques. Peggy Eckert, artist extraordinaire and author of *PJ's World — One Kids Memoir of Sorts*; Marie Trotignon, author of *Dancing in the Rain* and other books; Dianne MacDonald, author of *Growing up Electric* and other books; Barb Engle, author of *Gifts of the Tundra* and *Dr. D and Me*; Denise Yanega; Muriel Quint; and Gretchen Blanchard. They have sat through the readings of my book providing valuable insights, support and encouragement.

I thank my friends and family who have travelled with me to places and countries for the inspirational photographs. Thanks to Laura for her photographs of African figurines. Laurel for the night lights of LA and June for the lotus flower.

Thank you, my Tai Chi core group for providing a place for relaxation and keeping me grounded. I especially thank Gayle Colburn who painstakingly edited the entire manuscript and Paula Harms for her valuable direction and encouragement.

And last, but not least, I thank you, the reader for your interest.

NAMASTE

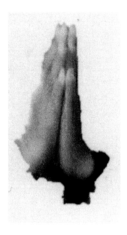

Permissions Credits

Every attempt has been made to comply with copyright requirements.

I acknowledge gratefully the following who have graciously allowed the reprint of their material through personal communication (email /phone).

1. Michael Modzelewski—*Inside Passage*; *Wild Life*
2. Edgar Mitchell—*The Way of the Explorer*, Career Press, 2008
3. Gloria Burgess—*Journey of the Rose*; *Dare to Wear your Soul on the Outside*, Jossey Bass, 2008
4. Ronald Potter-Efron—*Healing the Angry Brain*, New Harbinger Publications, 2012
5. Roy Baumeister—*The Cultural Animal: Human Nature, Meaning, and Social Life*, Oxford University Press, 2005
6. Michael Scott—*The Alchemist*, Random House Press, 2007
7. Christiane Northrup, MD—*The Wisdom of Menopause*, Bantam Books, 2012
8. Richard Dawkins—*The Selfish Gene*, Clays Ltd., 1976
9. Steven Pinker—*How the Mind Works*, W. W. Norton and Co., 1997

10. Gloria Steinem—*My Life on the Road*, Random House, 2015

11. Gregory Orr—*Concerning the Book That is the Body of the Beloved*, Copper Canyon Press, 2005

12. Peter McIntyre—*Kakahi New Zealand*, A.H. & A.W. Reed, 1972

13. C. Joybell C.—*Conversation of Dragons*, Vade Mecum, 2013

14. Savannah Page—*A Sister's Place*, Lake Union Publishing, 2015

15. Marianne Williamson—*A Return to Love*, Harper Collins, 1992